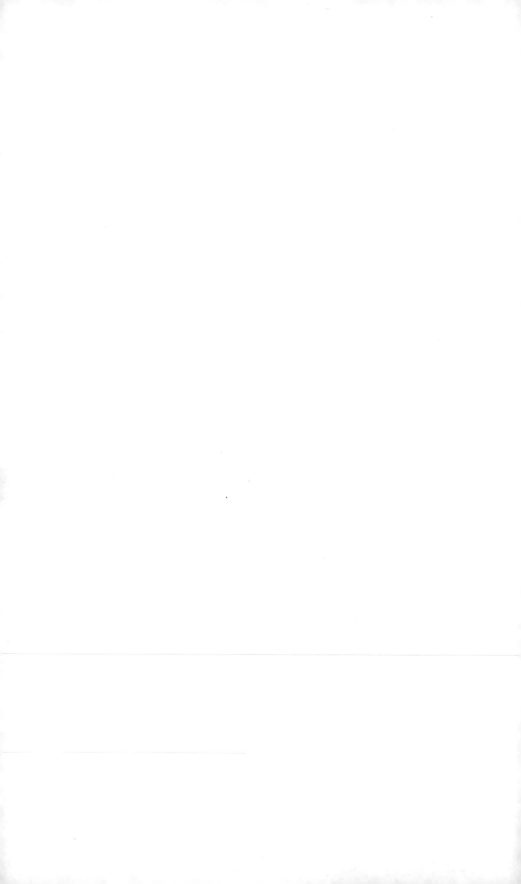

EPIDEMIOLOGIC PRINCIPLES AND FOOD SAFETY

EPIDEMIOLOGIC PRINCIPLES AND FOOD SAFETY

Edited by
Tamar Lasky

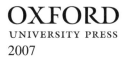

OXFORD
UNIVERSITY PRESS
2007

To my mother, Miriam

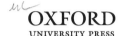

OXFORD
UNIVERSITY PRESS

Oxford University Press, Inc., publishes works that further
Oxford University's objective of excellence
in research, scholarship, and education.

Oxford   New York
Auckland   Cape Town   Dar es Salaam   Hong Kong   Karachi
Kuala Lumpur   Madrid   Melbourne   Mexico City   Nairobi
New Delhi   Shanghai   Taipei   Toronto

With offices in
Argentina   Austria   Brazil   Chile   Czech Republic   France   Greece
Guatemala   Hungary   Italy   Japan   Poland   Portugal   Singapore
South Korea   Switzerland   Thailand   Turkey   Ukraine   Vietnam

Published by Oxford University Press, Inc.
198 Madison Avenue, New York, New York 10016

www.oup.com

Oxford is a registered trademark of Oxford University Press

Library of Congress Cataloging-in-Publication Data
Epidemiologic principles and food safety / edited by Tamar Lasky.
p. ; cm.
Includes bibliographical references.
ISBN 978-0-19-517263-8
1. Food—Safety measures.   2. Epidemiology.   3. Food supply.   4. Food—Toxicology.
I. Lasky, Tamar.
[DNLM: 1. Food Contamination—prevention & control.   2. Epidemiologic Studies.
3. Food Handling—methods. WA 701 E64 2006]
RA1258.E65 2006
363.19'26—dc22   2006021979

9 8 7 6 5 4 3 2 1

Printed in the United States of America
on acid-free paper

FOREWORD

Food is much more than personal fuel—food creates community. We welcome friends and family into our homes with a meal. We celebrate important occasions with feasts. We carry food to those in mourning. We receive food as daily comfort. We don't think of food as a risk.

But there is risk.

When we consider factors that spread disease, ticks or rats spring to mind more quickly than scrambled eggs or a juicy hamburger. What could be more wholesome than those fresh sprouts at the salad bar? But foods bring risk, as this book bluntly reminds us. In the United States alone, millions are diagnosed each year with food poisoning, with 325,000 affected so severely that they require hospitalization. (Many thousands of others probably go undiagnosed.) While treatments are usually effective, food poisoning in the United States kills more than a thousand people annually.

The problems of food safety are not only serious—they are growing. Two crucial factors in this unfolding story are the increasingly industrialized production of food and the emergence of new infectious agents.

"Industrialization" of foods refers to a range of innovations in food production, preservation, and transportation that radically changed eating habits during the twentieth century. For the first time in human history, seasonal foods became available year-round. Commercially prepared foods took precedence over home-made. Food of all sorts became cheap.

As the industrialization of food continues to expand in the twenty-first century, new problems are emerging. Consider the complex networks by which food is distributed. The contamination of a prepared food in one factory can sicken hundreds of people in widely separated areas, concealing both the outbreak and its source. Globalization and the expansion of world trade further complicate epidemiologic detective work—an outbreak of food poisoning in Canada may trace back to an abattoir in Argentina or a greenhouse in South Africa.

A second major factor in food safety has been the emergence of new infectious diseases. Diseases carried by foods are part of a larger picture of emerging infections. Among the emerging food-borne infectious agents, the prion may be the most fascinating. Prions are the cause of such diseases as scrapie and bovine spongiform encephalopathy ("mad cow" disease). While prions are not life forms by conventional definition, they slowly catalyze lethal reactions in our food animals—and in us. Epidemiologists made some of the key observations on the infectious nature of prion diseases, and the tools of epidemiology will be necessary to monitor the future impact of these diseases.

Infectious agents are not our only worry. With industrialization comes an increased reliance on pesticides, leading to more pesticide exposures for those handling and eating food, with the potential for producing subtle and long-term problems. The ubiquity and chronic nature of pesticide exposures, together with their potential to produce diverse health effects, make their study by epidemiologists particularly challenging.

In coming to grips with new problems, epidemiologists have the advantage of new tools. Better integration and monitoring of medical information systems allow earlier detection of suspicious clusters of acute infections. Once identified, such clusters can be traced with molecular genetic assays that allow the "fingerprinting" of specific strains of organisms, and thus the precise identification of cases. Once an outbreak has been identified, public health actions may be required that cross national borders. The swift international response to the SARS (severe acute respiratory syndrome) epidemic has shown that effective cross-border interventions are possible.

Meanwhile, the public is becoming more aware of the emerging problems of food-borne diseases and the hidden costs of our cheap food. The essays of Wendell Berry bear witness to the ecologic virtues embodied in the small farm and lost with industrialized farming. Community farmers' markets are thriving as people rediscover the benefits of locally grown foods. Even so, these are small drops compared with the vast ocean of agribusiness. The spectrum of food-borne illnesses is increasingly complex, and the economic and social consequences are ever more far-reaching.

In this volume, experts from a range of disciplines address the problems of food safety in a scholarly and informative way. Chapters address how food safety has evolved over the years, the various ways in which food can become contaminated, and the use of epidemiologic methods to understand and control food-borne illness. With an insider's understanding of how the U.S. public health system works to prevent food-borne illness, this book is directed toward those with an interest in public health. Make no mistake: this topic should be compelling to anyone who eats.

Allen J. Wilcox

PREFACE

Epidemiology has long played a critical role in investigating outbreaks of food-borne illness and in identifying the microbial pathogens associated with such illness. In the past, epidemiologists were the detectives who would track down the guilty culprit—the food vehicle carrying the pathogen, as well as the fateful errors that resulted in contamination or multiplication of pathogens. Today, epidemiologists continue to investigate food-borne outbreaks, but epidemiologists also have a role in policy formation and outbreak prevention. By accumulating information across outbreaks, and for cases of food-borne illness not associated with a specific outbreak, epidemiologists can apply methods developed for the study of chronic diseases (e.g., heart disease or cancer) to identify points for intervention, inform risk assessors and policy makers, identify risk factors, and assess the contribution of steps along the farm-to-table continuum to the overall burden of food-borne disease.

Although epidemiologists working in food safety are primarily concerned with infectious agents, and must draw on methods developed within infectious disease epidemiology, they also must often draw on methods developed within chronic disease epidemiology. This intertwining of two strands of epidemiology may require the reader to adapt methods that are not yet available at the time of this writing. In this book, we have attempted to identify areas that provide a challenge to epidemiology, areas in which more methodologic research is required to more fully benefit from the application of epidemiologic principles. In these areas, epidemiologic ideas are being applied in new ways, for example, surveillance for outbreaks, where the unit is not an individual but an entire outbreak, or case–control studies of unrelated cases (sometimes termed "sporadic") of an infectious illnesses caused by a specific pathogen. These new applications push at the edges of the current methodology and will require growth and development of epidemiologic thinking to meet the needs of food safety scientists.

This book should introduce the reader to some of the key concepts applicable to epidemiology in the food safety context, and should also introduce the reader to key disciplines relevant to any discussion regarding the maintenance of a safe food supply. Epidemiologists unfamiliar with food safety issues will gain a broad understanding of the outbreak investigation, economic and policy concerns, and points of intervention along the farm-to-table continuum: from the farm, through processing, to preparation and consumption. Food scientists unfamiliar with epidemiology will gain knowledge of key epidemiologic principles applied to food safety, such as surveillance and descriptive epidemiology, methodology for estimating data points required in risk assessment, and study designs for testing hypotheses regarding factors contributing to the overall occurrence of food-borne illness.

More than in any other field in epidemiology, food safety activities take place within government agencies at the local, state, national, and international levels. One consequence is that definitions, perspectives, and methodologies become consolidated within a particular government agency and, being part of government, become established in law. Food scientists from different agencies and levels of government may work with different definitions and concepts, and there is very little opportunity to exchange ideas or modify scientific thinking within the bureaucratic structure of a specific agency. In this book, scientists have attempted to describe issues and principles in a generic form that can be applied within or outside the United States, Canada, Europe, and the world and can be useful to government at local, state, and national levels. By attempting to be generic, it may contradict policies or procedures of specific government entities, and this might lead to a sense of disconnect for some readers. Those in specific government agencies need to follow their agency's approach; however, general scientific discussions need to move beyond the mission and constraints of specific government agencies. Thus, this book will be useful for general discussions but is not meant to be a manual or guide book for any specific government agency or activity. Similarly, the majority of examples in the book are drawn from the United States, but we have attempted to bring in examples of food safety epidemiology from Canada, the United Kingdom, Denmark, and other countries, as well as the international activities promoted by the World Health Organization. Again, we aimed to produce a book with applications to various settings but do not fully describe any specific national approach.

One word about Internet resources—as with many other areas, the Internet provides a range of resources for food safety scientists, from descriptions of pathogens and their symptoms, to access to the most recent recall information, statistics, legislation, data collection forms, and more. We have avoided providing an extensive number of web addresses because these addresses change rapidly, but any scientist, professor, student, or reader will need to use this book in combination with resources available on the web and will need to individualize their approach to the many Internet resources available. The focus of this book is on generic principles that will apply in the next 10–15 years or longer. We have also avoided providing tables or charts of materials that are readily available on the Internet and more easily updated on the Internet than in a book (e.g., lists of pathogens and symptoms).

Finally, this book contains very little about intentional contamination of the food supply or bioterrorism. Although maintenance of a safe food supply includes protection from intentional tampering, biosecurity draws on content and methodology from security, criminal, law enforcement, and similar fields, very much beyond the scope of this book. Although intentional contamination of food may result in outbreaks that appear similar to accidental contamination, and epidemiologists may be the first to investigate outbreaks of intentional contamination, resolution of the outbreak and prevention of future breaks in security fall on those specially trained in bioterrorism prevention. Epidemiologists and public health workers may be in a unique position to participate in surveillance for bioterrorism, but this is a specialized activity that requires in-depth discussion in a context outside this book.

ACKNOWLEDGMENTS

I am always grateful for having received a liberal arts education at Grinnell College in Iowa, where I was encouraged to explore different disciplines and to apply the highest standards of scholarship to all questions. I was equally fortunate in the graduate training that I received in the Department of Epidemiology at the School of Public Health at the University of North Carolina–Chapel Hill. The department was a nurturing environment that fostered scientific excellence as well as awareness of the social context for so many health issues.

Ruth Etzel opened the field of food safety to me by bringing me to the Food Safety and Inspection Service at the U.S. Department of Agriculture. She introduced me to the many issues related to food safety and, in particular, the federal government's role and responsibilities. Allan Wilcox responded to my interest by suggesting the symposium on food safety held at the EpiCongress 2000 and further encouraged me to put my thoughts on paper by asking me to write a commentary for the journal *Epidemiology*. The ideas first put forth in that essay developed into this book. I also thank the MPH students from George Washington University who worked with me while I was at the Department of Agriculture. In particular, Wenyu Sun and Rekha Holtry did work that used descriptive epidemiology to explore new questions in food safety.

The scientists who contributed chapters to this book were generous with their time, patience, and expertise, writing and rewriting chapters, explaining concepts to me when necessary, writing more when asked, suffering edits and cuts, and maintaining energy and interest over the three years of writing this book. Each is an expert in their area, and each permitted their areas of expertise to be condensed into a single chapter, painfully omitting many fine points and details.

Jeffrey House, at Oxford University Press, enthusiastically encouraged me to proceed with the book, and Carrie Pedersen carried on the work begun by Jeffrey, with professionalism and genuine interest. She was assisted by Regan Hofmann and others in production of this book.

My children, Daphne and David, used reverse psychology to encourage me to write this book. Although they both learned to pronounce "bovine spongiform encephalopathy" relatively early in life, they have found the subject rather unglamorous. I thank them for reminding me of the world outside of public health and food safety, and the need to keep in perspective concerns about food safety.

CONTENTS

CONTRIBUTORS

Captain Sean Altekruse, DVM,
  MPH, PhD
U.S. Public Health Service
Assigned to Food Safety and Inspec-
  tion Service
U.S. Department of Agriculture
Washington, DC

Steven A. Anderson, PhD, MPP
Center for Biologics Evaluation and
  Research
U.S. Food and Drug Administration
Rockville, MD

Leila Barraj, DsC
Exponent, Inc.
Washington, DC

Luenda E. Charles, PhD, MPH
Centers for Disease Control and
  Prevention
National Institute for Occupational
  Safety and Health
Morgantown, WV

Sherri B. Dennis, PhD
Center for Food Safety and Applied
  Nutrition
U.S. Food and Drug Administration
Washington, DC

Captain Charles Higgins, MSEH,
  REHS
U.S. Public Health Service
Assigned to National Park Service,
  U.S. Department of the Interior
Washington, DC

James C. Kile, DVM, MPH, Diplomate ACVPM
Food Safety and Inspection Service
U.S. Department of Agriculture
Omaha, NE

Tamar Lasky, PhD
Associate Professor
College of Pharmacy
University of Rhode Island
Kingston, RI

Ritha Naji, MD
Saginaw VA Hospital,
Saginaw, MI

Tanya Roberts, PhD
Economic Research Service
U.S. Department of Agriculture
Washington, DC

A. Mahdi Saeed, DVM, MPH, PhD
Professor of Epidemiology and Public
Health
Department of Epidemiology
Michigan State University
East Lansing, MI

Nga L. Tran, DrPH, MPH
Exponent, Inc.
Washington, DC

EPIDEMIOLOGIC PRINCIPLES AND FOOD SAFETY

1

INTRODUCTION AND BACKGROUND

Tamar Lasky

The knowledge that food can be used as a vehicle for agents causing illness and death is ancient. Skill in applying agents to foods with the intent to sicken and kill was highly developed in ancient civilizations, and one would surmise that the skill developed after observing deaths and illness following naturally occurring poisoning. Indeed, we might even infer that the method succeeded because it was indistinguishable from the relatively common event of naturally occurring food-borne illness. The range of contaminants and poisons found in foods has always been wide, and while many intentional poisonings may have appeared to be natural events, the reverse is also possible, that many natural events may have been mistakenly attributed to deliberate and intentional actions by ill wishers and/or to supernatural forces. Untangling the cause of a food-borne illness has never been easy.

The concept of a food-borne illness preceded the germ theory by thousands of years. Even without understanding the specifics of microbiology, people can readily comprehend that the safety of food depends on controlling the process of food production from growing plants and raising animals, through harvesting, slaughter, processing, and preparation—from farm to table. The sanitarian movements of the nineteenth century, spurred by reformist writers such as Upton Sinclair, coupled with an increased understanding of microbiology, led to a science-based public health approach to food safety that is not much more than 100 years old.

Taking an even broader view, much of human endeavor involves the struggle to produce, acquire, and preserve food. The ability to store and preserve food decreases the need to produce and acquire food continuously but is valuable only if it maintains food quality and safety. Thus, there is an inherent tension between food supply (and cost) and food safety. When food is scarce, we may accept food that is less fresh and of lower quality; when interventions to promote food safety are added to a production process, the cost of the product might increase. Until recently in human history, most people grew and produced some or all of their own food, maintaining control of the food they consumed and linking their livelihoods to the buying and selling of different food commodities. The importance of trade and commerce to national strength and well-being resulted in careful controls of food production and distribution, some of which were originally a response to trade concerns but were then been applied to food safety concerns, as well. For example, laws governing the measuring and weighing of grains and crops and the quality of products are found in most civilizations (a bushel of wheat, e.g., should contain a bushel of wheat, and not be diluted by other, cheaper grains or materials). Today, such laws can be used to recall products whose ingredients do not match their labels; although the laws stem from principles of fair business practices, they can be used to protect persons with allergies to specific ingredients and who require accurate food labeling.

The intertwining of economics with food safety and quality may be greater than in other areas of public health and epidemiology. Food is an international trade commodity; the export and import of foods affect international trade issues and government stability. Much of the world is without access to an adequate supply of food, and much of the world's food supply is grown by smaller and smaller fractions of the population. Although economic issues reverberate in other areas of public health, such as health care disparities, access to care, regulation of industry, the intertwining between food and economics is extremely tight.

The ability to preserve food decreases a community's dependence on daily harvest, slaughter, or milking of animals. Storage of grains may be the simplest form of food preservation, but other ancient methods include dehydration or drying, heating, freezing and cooling (in caves, with ice blocks, in the snow), fermentation (alcohol, pickling, cheeses, fermented dairy products), and chemical preservation (salt, spices, other chemicals). Methods varied in their practicality, depending on geography, climate, and availability of alternative food sources, and in their reliability, depending on the skill and knowledge of the preserver, climate, population density, and housing conditions. Until the nineteenth century, however, preserving and processing of foods took place in the home, village, and local community, and consumers may have had thorough acquaintance with the persons processing or selling the finished food products. This may have led to some kind of social accountability for product quality and some level of consumer confidence in the processed or preserved products.

With the industrial revolution, food preservation and processing were also industrialized, resulting in greater centralization of production, wider distribution of products, and fewer personal links between consumers and producers. In the 1790s in France, Nicolas Appert developed a method of submerging corked bottles of foods in boiling water, preserving the food sufficiently well that Napoleon awarded him a 12,000 franc prize—the technology was needed by Napoleon's armies, which were suffering from malnutrition and starvation. Bottles were replaced by "canisters" in 1810 when Peter Durand, an Englishmen, developed wrought-iron cans. Canning factories were established in 1812 in New York, in 1813 in England, and in 1821 in Boston, where William Underwood established America's oldest canning company.

In the early twentieth century, Clarence Birdseye developed a "Multiplate Quick Freeze Machine," and by 1925 he had established his frozen food business, beginning with frozen fish fillets and then proceeding to meats, poultry, fruits, and vegetables. Along with new methods for preserving foods, industrialization brought new methods for processing larger and larger volumes of foods. Upton Sinclair captured the industrial quality of the Chicago stockyards, as well as the food safety consequences, in his 1906 novel, *The Jungle*.

The dairy industry was one of the earliest to become centralized. The first regular shipment of milk by rail took place in 1841, from Orange County, New York, to New York City. The milk bottle was invented in 1884, and the automatic bottle filler and capper was patented in 1886. With centralization and industrialization came concerns about a milk-borne pathogen, tuberculosis. By 1890, tuberculin testing of dairy herds was introduced. This step is interesting because it emphasizes animal health as a point of intervention. To the present day, one of the voices in the food safety arena is that of veterinarians and agricultural scientists focusing on the elimination of pathogens from animal herds and flocks. European countries, in particular, have been successful in maintaining *Salmonella*-free flocks of chickens, for example.

Other approaches to ensuring safety of milk followed. In 1892, a certification program for milk was introduced in New Jersey; this approach encourages consumers to consider food safety in their buying decisions and is similar to a program used today to market certified pork products. Commercial pasteurizing machines were introduced in 1895, representing the technological approach to providing pathogen-free foods, and today, advocates of meat irradiation draw direct parallels with the introduction of milk pasteurization. In 1908, Chicago passed the first compulsory pasteurization law requiring pasteurization of milk except if it came from tuberculin-tested cows. This last represents a hybrid approach that in some ways is most typical of many food safety efforts.

The multiple approaches to preventing milk-borne tuberculosis continued for several decades. Passions reached a peak in Iowa, where the Iowa Supreme Court found a public health program testing cows for bovine tuberculosis to be constitutional. Farmers protested, particularly angry about the consequence of a positive tuberculin test: slaughter of the animal. Ultimately, Governor Dan Turner declared martial law in Cedar County, where farmers "were in an ugly mood," and called in the National Guard; veterinarians then continued with their tuberculin screening program (Black, 1996). The Iowa "Cow War" provides a clear example of intense viewpoints and conflicting interests surrounding food safety—agricultural, economic, public health, and the role of government.

The preceding example illustrates some key elements in the efforts to regulate food safety: local, state, and federal agencies are involved; multiple agencies at each level can become involved—health, agriculture, commerce, and even the military; and multiple approaches are taken. The Food and Drug Administration (FDA) and the U.S. Department of Agriculture (USDA) share responsibility for food safety at the national level, and the history of the FDA is highly interwoven with that of the USDA (Young 1981; Swann 1998).

In 1849, the FDA was located in the Chemical Laboratory of the Agricultural Division in the Patent Office of the Department of Interior (see table 1-1), and in 1862 it moved with the Chemical Division when the USDA was created. The separation from the USDA did not take place until 1940, and since 1980, the FDA has been part of the Department of Health and Human Services. Regulatory authority still resides at both the FDA and the USDA, creating an interesting political and legal environment for those regulating food safety, investigating food-borne illness, and preventing food-borne illness. To complicate matters further, food regulation at the FDA takes place alongside regulation of drugs and has developed in that context.

In 1906, Congress passed two major pieces of food safety regulation: the U.S. Pure Food and Drugs Act and the Meat Inspection Act. The U.S. Pure Food and Drugs Act attempted to protect safety by regulating product labeling. It forbade interstate commerce in adulterated or misbranded food and drugs. This meant that ingredients could not substitute for the food, conceal damage, pose a health hazard, or constitute a filthy or decomposed substance. The food or drug label could not be false or misleading. This was followed by the 1938 Food, Drug, and Cosmetic Act, which set standards for food products such as margarine, jams, tomato products, cereals, and many others (figure 1-1). Shortly after, in 1940, the FDA was moved out of the USDA, an agency devoted to the needs of farmers, to a new and independent agency, the Federal Security Agency. In 1953 the FDA was moved to the Department

TABLE 1-1   Designation and location of the FDA in the federal government

Year	Designation and Location	Statute
1839	Patent Office, Department of State	5 Stat. 353, 354
1849	Chemical Laboratory of the Agricultural Division in the Patent Office, Department of the Interior	9 Stat. 395
1862	Chemical Division, USDA	12 Stat. 387
1889	Chemical Division, USDA	25 Stat. 659
1890	Division of Chemistry, USDA	26 Stat. 282, 283
1901	Bureau of Chemistry, USDA	31 Stat. 922, 930
1927	Food and Drug Insecticide Administration, USDA	44 Stat. 976, 1002
1930	Food and Drug Administration, USDA	46 Stat. 392, 422
1940	FDA, Federal Security Agency	54 Stat. 1234, 1237
1953	FDA, Department of Health, Education, and Welfare	67 Stat. 631, 632
1979	FDA, Department of Health and Human Services	93 Stat. 668, 695

Source: Food and Drug Administration History Office.

of Health, Education, and Welfare, which in 1980 was reorganized as the Department of Health and Human Services.

The Meat Inspection Act was passed on the same day as the Pure Foods and Drug Act. It required inspection of animals before slaughter and inspection of carcasses, and it established cleanliness standards for slaughterhouses and processing plants. The 1957 Poultry Products Inspection Act passed similar legislation for poultry. Authority to regulate meat and poultry remained with the USDA even after the FDA was moved out of the USDA. Today, the FDA maintains regulatory authority for drugs and most foods, but the USDA maintains authority for meats and foods containing meats.

The human dimension of food-borne illness caught the public's attention with the story of "Typhoid Mary." in 1906, Mary Mallon worked as a cook for a wealthy family on Long Island, New York, and was identified as the point source of an outbreak of typhoid that affected 6 of the 11 people in the household (figure 1-2). George Soper, a sanitary engineer, published his report in the June 15, 1907, issue of the *Journal of the American Medical Association*. Mary Mallon did not recall having had even a mild case of typhoid and became incensed when Soper told her she was carrying and spreading the disease. The role of a food handler in the spread of food-borne illness is of special interest in the world of food safety. Food preparation, in restaurants, school cafeterias, catering establishments, and nursing homes and in the home, requires careful handling by the people preparing and serving the food. A broad range of illnesses can be transmitted from individuals to food and then to consumers of the food, resulting in isolated cases of illness, as well as outbreaks. While training of food workers for safe food-handling practices is

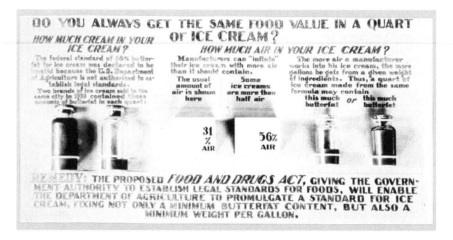

Figure 1-1. A poster linking the Food and Drug Act of 1938 to market concepts of fair trade. Source: Food and Drug Administration.

important, the health of the workers themselves is highly relevant to the safety of the food they handle and serve. Mary Mallon earned her living as a cook and continued to find positions as a cook until the New York City health inspector isolated her on North Brother Island (between the Bronx and Rikers Island), where she worked as a domestic. Although few would advocate such a drastic approach today, the essential conflict remains: many food workers report for work when ill with diarrhea or nausea, or carrying viruses such as hepatitis, and contaminate the food with which they work. Efforts to control the spread of illnesses from food workers (e.g., by requiring stool samples) are difficult and intrusive, and the cost of sick time to employer and employee discourages workers from staying home. The problem has barely been studied or addressed, but as consumers continue to eat more and more meals outside the home, concerns about the issue are sure to grow (e.g., 16% of all meals and snacks in 1977–1978 came from away-from-home sources, compared to 27% in 1995 [Lin et al. 1999]).

In many ways, it is surprising that food safety is of concern as we begin the twenty-first century. Developments in industry, processes such as pasteurization, canning, and refrigeration, stronger regulation of the food industry, and increased hygiene and packaging all have contributed to a decline in food-borne illness over much of the twentieth century. Figure 1-3 documents the steep decline in trichinosis (a food-borne parasite) over decades, until the 1990s when it approached zero cases per year. This accompanied an overall decline in mortality from infectious diseases in the United States and Europe, successful treatments for bacterial infections, and a growing concern with chronic diseases such as cancer and heart disease. Epidemiologists in the 1950s and

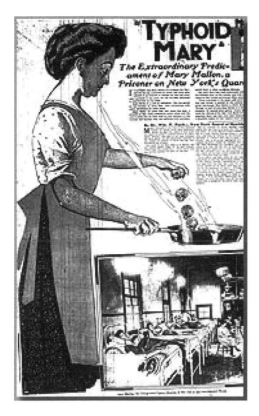

Figure 1-2. An illustration from the *New York American* (1909) calling attention to the typhoid cases linked to the cook Mary Mallon. Source: *Newsday.*

1960s expected to investigate food-borne outbreaks in the course of their careers, and epidemiology texts from those decades featured investigations of food-borne outbreaks in their teaching examples. By the 1970s and 1980s, infectious disease epidemiology no longer occupied center stage; epidemiology was engaged in the struggle to understand and control the epidemic of chronic diseases afflicting modern society, such as cancer and heart disease, and the dangers from occupational hazards and environmental exposures.

What changed between the 1980s and today? New infectious agents and diseases have emerged and been identified, beginning with human immunodeficiency virus (HIV, a retrovirus) and including bacterial pathogens such as *Campylobacter* and *E. coli* O157:H7 and prions such as that causing bovine spongiform encephalopathy (BSE, "mad cow" disease), thought to cause variant Creutzfeldt-Jacob disease in humans (figures 1-4, 1-5). Add to this the wider distribution of foods, greater amounts of food consumed outside the home, increased globalization and trading of foods, higher consumer expectations, increased antibiotic resistance, and a growing population of immune-deficient or

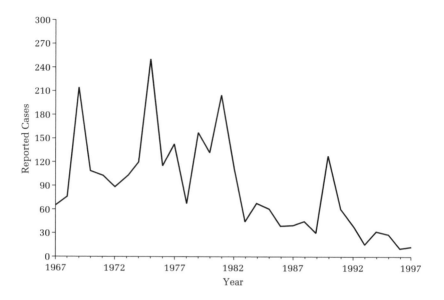

Figure 1-3. Trichinosis, by year, United States, 1967–1997. In 1997, a total of 13 trichinellosis (trichinosis) cases were reported, remaining at the lowest levels ever reported. When compared to rates several decades ago, the incidence of many food-borne illnesses has declined steeply, as is shown for trichinosis here. Trichinosis is a disease caused by *Trichinella*, a parasitic worm, associated with undercooked pork and wild game. Source: Centers for Disease Control and Prevention.

immune-suppressed individuals, and food-borne illness takes on new meaning. The popular press has fervently taken up food safety concerns: *Time*, *New Yorker*, *National Geographic*, and others have featured issues on the subject. Headlines incite a variety of fears and worries: "A World of Food Choices, and a World of Infectious Organisms" (*New York Times*, 2001), "Listeria Thrives in a Political Hotbed" (*New York Times*, 2002), "The Bug That Ate the Burger" (*Los Angeles Times*, 2001), "Clean Cutting Boards Are Not Enough: New Lessons in Food Safety" (*New York Times*, 2001), "An Outbreak Waiting to Happen" (*Washington Post*, 2001), "Denmark Sues EU Over Feta Cheese Ruling" (*New York Times*, 2002), "Consumer Groups Accuse U.S. of Negligence on Food Safety" (*New York Times*, 2002), "Food Safety Report Ignites Angry Debate" (*Washington Post*, 2002), "19 Million Pounds of Meat Recalled After 19 Fall Ill" (*New York Times*, 2002), and the classic but eternal "Hospital Flooded with Food Poisoning Cases after Church Supper" (*Boston Globe*, 2002).

Food safety is of critical concern as this new century begins, and epidemiologists have several roles in addressing the public health issues surrounding food safety. These include defining and measuring the burden of food-borne illness, describing the epidemiology of food-borne illness, investigating acute

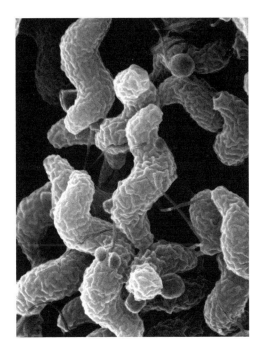

Figure 1-4. A scanning electron microscope image of corkscrew-shaped *Campylobacter jejuni* cells. The *Campylobacter* species were first identified in 1977 and is associated with gastroenteritis. Source: Agricultural Research Service.

outbreaks, identifying the factors contributing to non-outbreak illnesses, collecting and analyzing data for risk assessment, and working with interdisciplinary teams to develop and evaluate policies.

One feature of food-borne illness is that it is defined conceptually by the route of transmission—a legacy of its roots in infectious disease. However, one cannot always operationally distinguish infections that are food-borne from those transmitted by water, pets, sexual activity, or other routes of exposure. Salmonellosis acquired by toddlers mouthing objects from the floor is not a food-borne illness, and campylobacteriosis acquired from drinking contaminated water is not food-borne, yet such cases would be included in counts of infections that are "commonly food-borne." Furthermore, food-borne illnesses are not restricted to acute illnesses. There may be long latency periods, as with BSE. Finally, not all food-borne diseases are infectious. There may be allergic reactions to genetically modified plant proteins, or poisoning from chemical contaminants in food. The etiologic heterogeneity of "food-borne illness" makes it not entirely satisfactory as a disease category. This categorization does have value, however, from the point of view of intervention and prevention. For practical purposes, the logistics of maintaining a safe food supply requires attention to *all* illnesses that may be acquired through consumption of food. The range of pathogens leading to food-borne illness is described in chapter 2.

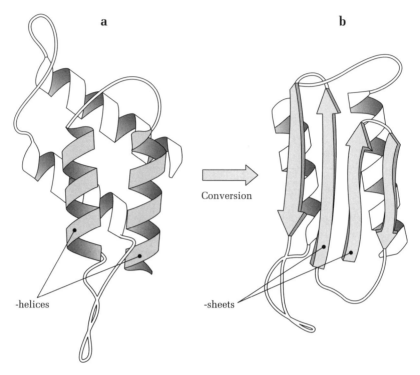

Figure 1-5. Prions, the agents associated with bovine spongiform encephalopathy (BSE), are proteins whose change in configuration leads to their infectivity. When meat from cattle with BSE is eaten, the prions can cause disease in humans. Source: Cold Spring Harbor Laboratory Press. Reprinted with permission of Cold Spring Harbor Laboratory Press.

Food-borne illness is closely identified with gastrointestinal illnesses, and the latter often serve as indicators of the burden of food-borne illness. Attempts have been made to estimate food-borne illness through the use of such indicator outcomes as "intestinal infectious diseases," self-reported diarrhea, or culture-confirmed cases of specific pathogens. Each approach (whether based on symptom or pathogen) is limited in its description of the complete picture of food-borne illness. When a case is defined by symptoms or laboratory culture, the case group will include non-food-borne cases—thus overestimating the burden of food-borne illness. On the other hand, many cases of food-borne illness are not reported; patients may decide not to seek care, doctors may choose not to collect specimens or order culture tests, and laboratories may not culture routinely for the pathogen in question. Data derived from clinical or surveillance sources may thus greatly underestimate the actual number of cases. Chapter 3 reviews efforts to measure the burden of food-borne illness, surveillance systems, and the descriptive epidemiology of food-borne illness.

The problem of definition goes beyond laboratory screening for common infectious agents. Food safety officials also need to be able to recognize unexpected events, such as those due to chemical contamination of food, long-term sequelae of infections, and reactions to genetically modified foods. These health events are not always considered in estimates of the burden of food-borne disease but may nonetheless consume public health and other resources. They have major consequences for industry and trade and receive a great deal of publicity. A good example is the task of keeping the meat supply free of prions that cause BSE. In the United States, there have been strenuous efforts to sample and test animals, restrict trade, regulate animal feed, and seize animals to prevent *any* occurrence of this food-borne illness. This public health program may have been taken for granted when it maintained a success rate of zero infected cows but seems inadequate after the identification of cases and a failure to keep BSE out of the United States. Highly successfully programs (maintaining low levels of illness) will consume public health resources and show little impact in health indicators (if they have reached zero, no further change is possible, yet the zero level must be maintained). A comprehensive approach to food-borne illness requires us to assess not only the illnesses spread by food but also the threats posed by potential illnesses. Only in this way can we measure our successes and the impact of dollars allocated to food safety.

Epidemiologists will play key roles in refining surveillance systems to include all food-borne conditions, adjust for factors that cause underestimates, separate food-borne cases from non-food-borne cases, and detect rare or unexpected events.

Two general approaches are taken to the study of food-borne illness. The first is used in an acute outbreak, when quick intervention may prevent further illness. This requires classic outbreak investigatory skills to identify the pathogen and the vehicle and source of contamination, and to control the specific outbreak. The second approach is to generalize beyond a specific outbreak to the universe of food-borne illness and thus identify measures that will lead to an overall lower number of outbreaks and an overall lower burden of food-borne illness. Chapter 4 reviews causal thinking, and ties together the approach taken when investigating acute outbreaks as well as aggregates of "sporadic" cases. Chapter 5 discusses dietary exposure assessment an area that draws heavily on work done by nutritionists, epidemiologists and dieticians, and is then critical to risk assessment.

Chapter 6 discusses investigation of outbreaks. In an acute outbreak, the main goal is to identify the source of exposure in order to prevent additional people from becoming ill. The reconstructed cohort method has been the primary approach used, particularly for outbreaks in which all exposed persons could be identified readily (e.g., the church picnic scenario). In recent years, investigators have also begun to use the case–control study design.

If the contamination originated on farms or during processing, steps can be taken to recall contaminated products from retailers and issue warnings to consumers. However, this requires identification of the food product by specific information (e.g., brand, lot, processing date, and sell-by date). A large part of the outbreak investigation may be dedicated to acquiring this detailed information. Investigators have painstakingly traced illnesses in disparate geographic locations to single-source products, to processing plants, or even to individual farms from which they originated. For example, an outbreak of *Shigella sonnei* in restaurants was traced to one lettuce-shredding plant, cases of hepatitis A were associated with fresh produce contaminated before distribution to restaurants, *Shigella flexneri* was traced to salad prepared at a central commissary of a restaurant chain, an outbreak of *Salmonella* was traced to cilantro grown on one farm, and an outbreak of *E. coli* O157:H7 was traced back to farms where 1% of the cattle tested positive for *E. coli* O157:H7 (Davis et al. 1988; Ostroff et al. 1990; Rosenblum et al. 1990; Dunn et al. 1995; Campbell et al. 2001). More information about agricultural practices, food production, and food processing can be found in chapters 10 and 11.

Pathogens can be introduced by food handlers through a broad range of improper handling practices; for example, an outbreak of *Salmonella* enteritis infection was attributed to a single employee (Hedberg et al. 1991). Home preparation can also be a danger; for example, an outbreak of *Salmonella* Typhimurium was associated with improper reheating of roast pork in individual homes (Gessner and Beller 1994). Chapter 11 describes how food handling introduces an additional layer of complexity in maintaining food safety. Proper food handling can eliminate risks associated with pathogens in some foods, while improper food handling can introduce pathogens not previously present or promote growth of pathogens already present. The association of code violations or failed health inspections with disease outbreaks has not been simple to quantify. Outbreaks have been reported at frequently penalized restaurants, and a case–control study in King County, Washington (Irwin et al. 1989), found a correlation between mean inspection score and reports of an outbreak. A second case–control study in Miami-Dade County, Florida (Cruz et al. 2001), did not find routine restaurant inspection violations to be predictive of food-borne outbreaks except for one critical violation, evidence of vermin. Epidemiologic research should be able to help identify practices that are most strongly predictive of food safety and thus provide a systematic basis for regulation and enforcement. Another approach to the problem of poor food handling has been taken by the Environmental Health Specialists Network, an initiative of the Centers for Disease Control and Prevention. This is an effort to describe the events and conditions that encourage improper food-handling practices (and outbreaks) at retail establishments. This reintroduces epidemiology to its old cousin, sanitarianism, in order to identify areas for intervention and prevention.

Acute outbreaks demand immediate attention, while in contrast, reduction of the overall levels of food-borne illness requires a comprehensive understanding of the contribution of many different factors to the aggregate group of food-borne cases. Several approaches have been taken to summarize information and generalize beyond individual outbreaks: (1) summaries across outbreak investigations, somewhat like a meta-analysis; (2) population-based case–control studies to identify behaviors, food groups, and other factors contributing to risk of food-borne illness; and (3) studies across restaurants and food service sites to identify environmental antecedents of improper food-handling practices. These approaches are discussed in chapter 8. In the second approach, researchers compare cases to controls with respect to eating habits, recalled dietary intake, and other factors such as owning pets, visiting farms, or traveling abroad. This is a fascinating example of a concept taken from chronic disease epidemiology and applied to infectious diseases. Ironically, the approach of studying multiple risk factors in chronic disease epidemiology was originally viewed as inconsistent with the concepts of causality that had been developed in infectious disease epidemiology. The adaptation of the population-based case–control study to the study of heterogeneous cases of food-borne illness may require more thought and attention to methodologic issues. Sophisticated statistical analysis is required to assess the interrelationship among variables such as education and social class, potential risk factors such as food-handling practices or eating in restaurants, and accompanying risk factors for non-food-borne acquisition of "commonly food-borne" pathogens (e.g., water supply or pet ownership). In particular, precise estimates of attributable risk associated with specific food groups or handling practices may require further work.

The food safety community has put forward the concept of the "farm-to-table continuum," emphasizing the importance of all stages of food production, transportation, and consumption in assuring food safety. We know from experience with individual outbreaks that contamination or improper handling at any step along the way can result in illness or death. The epidemiology of food-borne illness, which has historically been involved in well-contained individual outbreaks, now needs to integrate its work across many levels of food production, processing, and distribution. Sound policies on prevention of food-borne illness depend increasingly on risk assessment. This is true for policies at all levels of government, nationally and internationally. While risk assessment for environmental exposures has been undertaken for almost two decades, risk assessment for food safety policy is more recent, and the focus is somewhat different (Lammerding and Paoli 1997; Samet and Burke 1998; Samet et al. 1998). A major part of environmental risk assessment is hazard identification or hazard characterization—an assessment of the causal relationship between the exposure and diseases in question. In microbial food safety risk assessment, the causal agent is known. The pathogen in question is by definition a cause of disease. The unknown is the dose–response relationship, or a minimum "safe" dose. Human dose data are scarce. There is a wide range of potential doses that can be delivered with various foods, methods of preparation, cooking and storing temperatures, and so forth. Food safety risk assessment is often used to evaluate the impact of potential interventions, changes in production and processing, and regulations regarding food production and handling. Such models use the quantitative relation between dose and infection to estimate the number of cases potentially prevented by the proposed change in production practice or regulation. Chapter 9 describes risk assessment and food safety, and chapters 12 and 13 discuss economic and regulatory issues regarding epidemiology, risk assessment, and food safety.

The United States has experienced one reported outbreak of a food-borne illness caused by intentional contamination of food (Torok et al. 1997). In 1984, members of a religious commune deliberately contaminated salad bars in 10 restaurants in Oregon, resulting in 751 reported cases of *Salmonella* gastroenteritis. The possibility of intentional contamination has grown over the past decade, and epidemiologists along with the rest of the public health community have recently intensified their awareness of this issue. As mentioned above, malicious and intentional adulteration of food is an age-old method of murder. Current concerns about biosecurity reflect a renewed awareness of vulnerability when ingesting food and raise a wide range of questions well beyond the scope of this book and of epidemiology. While basic investigative epidemiologic skills will be necessary for identifying bioterrorism events and maintenance of a secure food supply, much of the know-how and methodology will come from law enforcement, law, defense, and other fields outside of epidemiology and public health. For the most part, these issues are beyond the scope of this book.

The focus here instead is on a new approach to epidemiology of food-borne illness that is broader and more comprehensive than the outbreak investigations of the past. This new approach has its roots in the study of infectious disease but draws on other branches of epidemiology. The dividing line between chronic and infectious disease epidemiology has been eroding in all areas of epidemiology. Food-borne illness is one more example of the blurring of this distinction, as newly discovered agents carried in food are implicated in diseases of long latency. The chapters in this book show how methods from both infectious disease epidemiology and chronic disease epidemiology can be used to identify immediate causes of acute outbreaks, as well as primary causes of the overall societal burden of food-borne illness.

References

Black, Neal (1996). Tuberculosis. In *Animal Health: A Century of Progress*. Richmond, VA, U.S. Animal Health Association: 32–37.

Black, Neal (1998). Tuberculosis. In *Animal Health: A Century of Progress*. Richmond, VA, U.S. Animal Health Association: 22–37

Campbell, J. V., J. Mohle-Boetani, et al. (2001). An outbreak of Salmonella serotype Thompson associated with fresh cilantro. *J Infect Dis* 183(6): 984–987.

Cruz, M. A., D. J. Katz, and J. A. Suarez. (2001). An Assessment of the Ability of Routine Restaurant Inspections to Predict Food-Borne Outbreaks in Miami-Dade County, Florida. *Am J Public Health* 91(5): 821–823.

Davis, H., J. P. Taylor, et al. (1988). A shigellosis outbreak traced to commercially distributed shredded lettuce. *Am J Epidemiol* 128(6): 1312–1321.

Dunn, R. A., W. N. Hall, et al. (1995). Outbreak of *Shigella flexneri* linked to salad prepared at a central commissary in Michigan. *Public Health Rep* 110(5): 580–586.

Federal Food, Drug and Cosmetic Act, 21 U.S.C. Sec. 301 (1938).

Federal Meat Inspection Act, 21 U.S.C. Sec. 601 (1906).

Gessner, B. D., and M. Beller. (1994). Protective effect of conventional cooking versus use of microwave ovens in an outbreak of salmonellosis. *Am J Epidemiol* 139: 903–909.

Hedberg, C. W., K. E. White, et al. (1991). An outbreak of *Salmonella* enteritidis infection at a fast-food restaurant: implications for foodhandler-associated transmission. *J Infect Dis* 164(6): 1135–1140.

Irwin, K., J. Ballard, et al. (1989). Results of routine restaurant inspections can predict outbreaks of foodborne illness: The Seattle-King County experience. *Am J Public Health* 79(5): 1678–1679.

Lammerding, A. M., and G. M. Paoli. (1997). Quantitative risk assessment: an emerging tool for emerging foodborne pathogens. *Emerg Infect Dis* 3(4): 483–487.

Lin, B.-H., E. Frazao, et al. (1999). Away-from-home foods increasingly important to quality of American diet. Economic Research Service, U.S. Department of Agriculture, Washington, DC.

Ostroff, S. M., P. M. Griffin, et al. (1990). A statewide outbreak of *Escherichia coli* O157:H7 infections in Washington State. *Am J Epidemiol* 132(2): 239–247.

Rosenblum, L. S., I. R. Mirkin, et al. (1990). A multifocal outbreak of hepatitis A traced to commercially distributed lettuce. *Am J Public Health* 80(9): 1075–1079.

Samet, J. M., and T. A. Burke. (1998). Epidemiology and risk assessment. In *Applied Epidemiology: Theory to Practice* (R. C. Brownson and D. B. Petitti, eds.). New York, Oxford University Press: 137–176

Samet, J. M., R. Schattner, et al. (1998). Epidemiology and risk assessment. *Am J Epidemiol* 148: 929–936.

Swann, J. P. (1998). Food and Drug Administration. In *A Historical Guide to the US Government* (G. T. Kurian, ed.). New York, Oxford University Press: 248–254.

Torok, T. J., R. V. Tauxe, et al. (1997). A large community outbreak of salmonellosis caused by intentional contamination of restaurant salad bars. *JAMA* 278(5): 389–395.

Young, J. H. (1981). The long struggle for the 1906 law. *FDA Consumer* 15(5).

2

INFECTIOUS AGENTS

A. Mahdi Saeed and Ritha Naji

Food can be contaminated by microbial organisms as well as by chemicals and physical agents. Because all our food comes from plants and animals, exposure of food sources to the microorganisms living in the air, water, and soil is inevitable. Plant foods will retain some pathogens found in the water and soil, and animals raised for food can be infected by pathogens transmitted by insects, rodents, water, and exposure to other animals. Food-borne pathogens include bacteria, parasites and protozoa, viruses, and prions. Each of these groups of pathogens is found in nature and can cause illness when proper care is not taken to clean and eliminate pathogens from foods. Most pathogens are living organisms and named, like other living organisms, by genus and species. Some examples of the taxonomies are presented in table 2-1.

Over the past three decades, several new pathogens—including bacterial, parasitic, viral, and prion—have been discovered. The emergence of newly recognized infectious diseases is one of the factors that brings the issue of food-borne illness back into the arena of public concern, as methods for diagnosis, testing, and treatment are developed in response. The most common food-borne pathogens are described below, along with specific examples, clinical symptoms of disease, and diagnostic and laboratory testing procedures. This is followed by a short discussion of toxins produced by microorganisms.

TABLE 2-1   Examples of pathogen taxonomies

Kingdom	Family	Genus	Species
Monera	Campylobacteraceae	*Campylobacter*	
	Enterobacteriaceae	*Escherichia*	
		Listeria	
		Salmonella	
	Enterobacteriaceae	*Shigella*	
		Yersinia	
Protista	Cryptosporidiidae	*Cryptosporidium*	
		Cyclospora	
	Hexamitidae	*Giardia*	
		Toxoplasma	
	Trichinellidae	*Trichinella*	
Viruses (sometimes included in Monera)	Picornaviridae	*Hepatovirus*	*Hepatitis A*
	Caliciviridae	*Calicivirus*	*Norwalk virus*

Bacteria

Both aerobic and anaerobic bacteria can cause food-borne illness. The most commonly recognized food-borne bacterial pathogens are *Campylobacter*, *Escherichia coli*, *Listeria*, *Salmonella*, *Shigella*, *Vibrio*, and *Yersinia*.

Campylobacter

Campylobacters were first isolated in 1972 by a clinical microbiologist in Belgium from stool samples of patients with diarrhea (Kist, 1985). In the 1970s, development of selective growth media helped laboratories to isolate campylobacters from patients' stool specimens. *Campylobacter* species are currently among the most common human pathogens, causing large numbers of cases of acute bacterial enteritis in most parts of the world (Nachamkin, 2002; Fisher et al 2006). Symptoms of patients with laboratory-confirmed infections include bloody diarrhea, fever, and abdominal cramping (Blaser, 1997).

Escherichia coli

Escherichia coli are ubiquitous gram-negative bacteria and naturally inhabit the intestines of humans and most warm-blooded animals without causing illness (figure 2-1). However, six classes of pathogenic *E. coli* cause severe and sometimes fatal gastroenteritis in humans (Kaper, 2005):

- Enteroaggregative *E. coli*, which express an aggregative pattern of interaction with tissue culture cells such as Hep-2 cells maintained in tissue culture medium Enterohemorrhagic *E. coli*, which are associated with hemorrhagic colitis and hemolytic uremic syndrome

- Enteroinvasive *E. coli*, which invade the intestinal epithelium in a manner similar to that of *Shigella*
- Enteropathogenic *E. coli*, which mediate their pathogenic effect via attachment to and effacing of the intestinal epithelial cells
- Enterotoxigenic *E. coli*, which liberate several classes of enterotoxins (STa, STb) that mediate the diarrheal disease they cause in humans and animals

Of these classes, enterohemorrhagic *E. coli* O157:H7 is the most serious and produces one or more potent toxins that cause severe damage to the lining of the intestine. *Escherichia coli* O157:H7 was first recognized as a cause of illness in 1982 during an outbreak of severe bloody diarrhea that was traced to contaminated hamburgers (Tuttle et al., 1999). Infection often leads to bloody diarrhea and, in rare instances, can be followed by hemolytic uremic syndrome (figure 2-2). Consumption of ground beef, lettuce, raw cider, raw milk, and untreated water has been implicated in outbreaks, and person-to-person transmission is well documented. The organism can be found on a small number of cattle farms and can live in the intestines of healthy cattle. Meat can become contaminated during slaughter, and organisms can be thoroughly mixed into beef when it is ground.

Listeria

Of the several species of genus *Listeria*, the two of human pathogenic significance are *L. monocytogenes* and *L. ivanovii*. *Listeria monocytogenes* is a

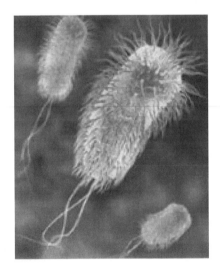

Figure 2-1. Microbial pathogens include bacteria, viruses, parasites, and prions. This figure shows the bacterium *E. coli* O157:H7. Source: Center for Meat Process Validation, University of Wisconsin-Madison.

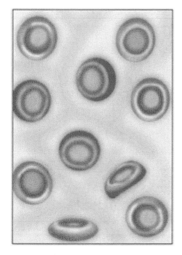

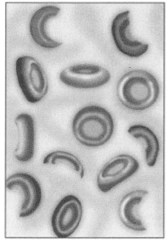

Figure 2-2. Bacterial toxins cause disease by damaging human cells. Hemolytic uremic syndrome develops when toxins damage blood platelets, as illustrated by these drawings (left, healthy cells; right, damaged cells). Such toxins are produced by *E. coli* O157. Source: National Institutes of Health.

gram-positive food-borne pathogen that has been implicated in several food poisoning epidemics. It is ubiquitous in nature and can be isolated from the gastrointestinal tract of several animals and up to 5% of healthy humans. The bacterium usually causes septicemia and meningitis in patients with compromised immune function. It also causes encephalitis, which is an inflammation of the brain. *Listeria monocytogenes* are facultative intracellular bacteria that can multiply in environments totally devoid of host cells. There are 13 known serotypes of *L. monocytogenes*. Of these, serotype 4b strains cause more than half of the listeriosis cases worldwide (Aarnisalo et al., 2003, whereas most strains found in food are serotype 1/2a and 1/2b (Wallace et al., 2003). Contaminated refrigerated ready-to-eat foods are of particular concern since such products typically are not heated prior to consumption.

Salmonella

Salmonella are motile, gram-negative, rod-shaped bacteria of the family Enterobacteriaceae. The genus is named after Daniel E. Salmon, who first isolated the organisms in 1884 from porcine intestine. *Salmonella* are common in the gastrointestinal tracts of mammals, reptiles, birds, and insects. All salmonellae are grouped into a single overarching species, *Salmonella enterica*, which is divided into seven subgroups (I–VII) based on DNA homology and host range. Most of the salmonellae that are pathogenic in humans belong to a single subgroup (subgroup I) and can be further categorized into more than 2,500 serovars, or serotypes, based on their immunodominant somatic O, surface Vi, and flagellar H antigens. In 2000, the 10 most frequently isolated *Salmonella* strains causing human disease among the 4,095 isolates serotyped and reported to the U.S. Centers for Disease Control and Prevention (CDC) were as follows: 982 (24%) were serotype Typhimurium, 403 (10%) were serotype Enteritidis, 362 (9%) were serotype Newport, 284 (7%) were serotype Heidelberg, and 231 (6%) were serotype Muenchen; 405 (10%) of *Salmonella* isolates were untyped. Based on the Preliminary FoodNet Data on the Incidence of Infection with Pathogens Transmitted Commonly Through Food—10 States, United States, 2005, *Salmonella* decreased 9% (CI = 2%–15%). Although *Salmonella* incidence decreased overall, of the five most common *Salmonella* serotypes, only the incidence of *S.* Typhimurium decreased significantly (42% [CI = 34%–48%]). The estimated incidence of *S.* Enteritidis increased 25% (CI = 1%–55%), *S.* Heidelberg increased 25% (CI = 1%–54%), and *S.* Javiana increased 82% (CI = 14%–191%). The estimated incidence of *S.* Newport increased compared with the baseline, but the increase was not statistically significant (CDC 2006).

    Salmonella are categorized as typhoidal or nontyphoidal. Typhoidal *Salmonella* serovars include *Salmonella* Typhi, and *Salmonella* Paratyphi, whose incidence started declining since the 1960s and nontyphoidal *Salmonella* include more than 2,500 serotypes. While reservoirs of typhoidal *Salmonella* are found in humans, reservoirs of the nontyphoidal *Salmonella* are widespread, found in the intestinal tracts of domestic and wild animals, in soil, and in water. Of increasing concern is the number of *Salmonella* strains observed in animal reservoirs and in samples taken after human illness and food-borne outbreaks that have developed resistance to antimicrobial drugs, for example, *Salmonella* Typhimurium DT104 and *Salmonella* Newport.

    Salmonella infection may lead to any of three distinct syndromes: gastroenteritis, typhoid (enteric) fever, or focal disease. Infection with nontyphoidal salmonellae usually causes enterocolitis similar to that caused by other bacterial enteric pathogens. Nausea, vomiting, and diarrhea occur within 6–48 hours after ingestion of contaminated food or drink. In most cases, stools are loose and bloodless. Salmonellae may rarely cause large-volume cholera-like diarrhea or may be associated with tenesmus. The diarrhea is typically self-limiting and resolves within 3–7 days. While infection with S, Typhi and S. paratyphi are very infrequent , an initial transient diarrhea may occur. However, infection with these serotypes are associated with abdominal pain and either constipation or recurrent diarrhea in approximately 40% of cases. Fever, abdominal cramping, chills, headache, and myalgia are also common. Cases of endocarditis with *Salmonella* infections (*Salmonella* Typhimurium or *Salmonella* Choleraesuis) have been reported. *Salmonella* pneumonia is rare in the absence of other illnesses. Individuals with urinary calculi or obstruction of the urinary tract and individuals receiving immunosuppressive therapy have been reported with urinary tract *Salmonella* infections. Cases of meningitis have been reported in infants and children.

Salmonella Enteritidis emerged during the early 1970s and has been associated with consumption of inadequately cooked eggs and egg-containing foods (Saeed et al 1999), 1999). This emerging serotype surpassed *Salmonella* Typhimurium during 1993 and is still the most common *Salmonella* serotype isolated from human and nonhuman sources in several European countries.

Shigella

Shigella is an invasive pathogen that is closely related to *E. coli*. Four species, *S. dysenteriae*, *S. flexneri*, *S. boydii*, and *S. sonnei*, are most frequently associated with shigellosis. Among 2,529 isolates obtained from travelers with diarrhea, *S. sonnei* was the most common serogroup (67%), followed by *S. flexneri* (26%), *S. boydii* (5%), and *S. dysenteriae* (3%) (Ekdahl and Andersson, 2005). Shigellosis can manifest as diarrhea accompanied by fever, tiredness, watery or bloody diarrhea, nausea and vomiting, and abdominal pain. These symptoms usually begin within 2 days of being exposed to *Shigella* and usually are gone within 5–7 days. *Shigella* is highly infectious, needing only 10–100 bacteria to transmit cause an infection in humans. *Shigella* is primarily transmitted through fecal–oral contact and is readily transmitted by food handlers. In some populations, it has come to be recognized as a sexually transmitted illness. People with shigellosis usually recover completely, but certain strains of *S. dysenteriae* type 1 produce Shiga toxin and can lead to life-threatening hemolytic uremic syndrome, the same complication that develops in some cases of infection with *E. coli* O157:H7.

Vibrio vulnificus

First reported in 1979, *Vibrio vulnificus* has emerged as one the most virulent food-borne pathogen in the United States (Blake et al., 1979). *Vibrio vulnificus* infections resulting from the ingestion of raw or undercooked seafood could lead to septicemic cases with a fatality rate of 50–60%. Symptoms occur within 16–38 hours and include fever, chills, a decrease in blood pressure, and the development of secondary lesions, typically on the legs. These lesions begin as fluid-filled blisters and progress to extensive destruction of muscle tissue, frequently requiring amputation of the affected limb. The infection ends fatally in half of the individuals with advanced cases that do not receive appropriate treatment. Most cases occur in individuals with underlying immunocompromising diseases or diseases such as liver cirrhosis, chronic hepatitis, and hemochromatosis that lead to elevated serum iron levels (Oliver and Kaper 2001).

Yersinia

Yersinia enterocolitica resembles other common Enterobacteriaceae but can grow at both 25°C and 37°C within 48 hours particularly on selective media such as cefsulodin-irgasan-novobiocin (CIN) agar. Researchers have developed two biotyping systems that led to the identification of 34 serotypes and five biotypes. The serotypes that most clearly are pathogenic to humans include serotypes O:3, O:5, O:27, O:8, O:9, and O:13. Accurate identification of pathogenic strains requires consideration of both the biotype and the serotype because multiple cross-reacting O factors can occur in some strains (Hinrek and Cheasty, 2006)

 Yersinia enterocolitica can cause a variety of symptoms depending on the age of the person infected. Common symptoms in children are fever, abdominal pain, and diarrhea. In older children and adults, right-sided abdominal pain and fever may be confused with appendicitis. The major animal reservoir for *Y. enterocolitica* strains that cause human illness is pigs. Infection is acquired by eating contaminated food, especially pork products, particularly raw pork intestines (chitterlings). Contaminated unpasteurized milk or untreated water can also transmit the infection to humans. The infection can be transmitted from person to person due to inadequate hygiene.

Laboratory Tests for Bacterial Pathogens

When bacterial causes are suspected in food-borne illnesses, stools from clinical cases are collected and analyzed to identify the specific pathogen. Stools are typically collected and transported to the laboratory under refrigerated conditions using a transport medium to stabilize the suspected bacterial entities and prevent gross overgrowth by bacterial contaminants. In addition to epidemiologic data suggesting an association with a specific food source, the diagnosis of most food-borne bacterial pathogens is confirmed when the suspected bacteria is found in a stool culture or is isolated from the contaminated food. Bacterial entities are identified by their behavior on specific isolation media; by their biochemical profiles using methods such as miniaturized kits, and serological confirmation using group and individual-specific antisera confirms the identity of the isolates. Some of the isolates, such as the hemolytic uremic *E. coli*, are tested for verotoxin production by using molecular probes to identify specific genes that are associated with the verotoxins. Molecular subtyping of bacterial isolates by characterization of nucleic acids has helped epidemiologic investigations of outbreaks of food-borne illness (Tenover et al., 1995; Lee et al., 1998).

Several methods for identifying restriction-fragment-length polymorphisms (RFLPs) on chromosomal DNA have been developed, and molecular subtyping has become an essential component of epidemiologic investigations of infectious diseases (Ribot et al., 2001). During the investigation of several *E. coli* O157:H7 outbreaks caused by contaminated hamburgers served in a fast-food restaurant chain in the western United States, the CDC laboratories applied pulsed-field gel electrophoresis to characterize clinical and food isolates of *E. coli* O157:H7, demonstrating its utility in outbreak investigations (figure 2-3). Subtyping activities and standardized molecular subtyping methodology were then transferred to several states' public health laboratories to enable timely subtyping of clinical and food isolates. Results of subtyping activities were frequently useful to epidemiologists in the course of outbreak investigations. Use of standardized subtyping methods allows isolates to be compared from different parts of the country, helping to identify outbreaks not readily recognizable by other means. These results were valuable in the recognition of national and international outbreaks attributable to a common source of infection, particularly those in which cases are geographically separated. An example of such an outbreak is the simultaneous outbreaks of Escherichia coli O157:H7 infection in Michigan and Virginia in June and July 1997, which were independently associated with eating alfalfa sprouts grown from the same seed lot. The outbreak strains in Michigan and Virginia were indistinguishable by PFGE molecular subtyping methods (CDC, MMWR August 1997).

Parasites and Protozoa

Parasites such as *Cryptosporidium*, *Cyclospora*, and *Giardia* are abundant in the environment and in water sources and can readily contaminate foods and produce. Some other parasites live in intermediate hosts, such as the encysted forms of *Toxoplasma gondii* in pigs and the encysted larval stage of *Taenia saginata* in cattle and *Taenia solium* and *Trichinella spiralis* in pigs. Humans become infected when they consume raw or inadequately cooked meats that containing these encysted stages of the parasites. Parasitic species may contaminate water used for growing or washing fruits and vegetables at the farm or processing points, which can lead to outbreaks.

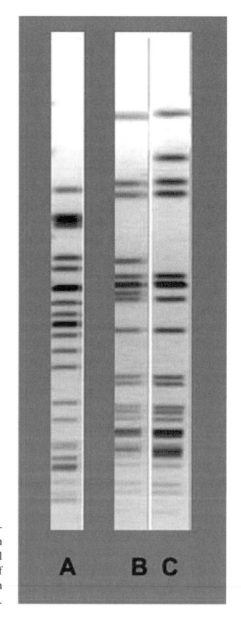

Figure 2-3. Pulsed-field gel electrophoresis typing of bacteria relies on patterns of bands that separate in a gel based on the weights of the fragments of the proteins. Source: Public Health Agency of Canada.

Entamoeba histolytica

This protozoal parasite causes amebiasis characterized by dysentery, stomach pain, bloody stools, and fever. *Entamoeba histolytica* can invade the liver, forming an abscess, and can even spread to the lungs or brain. However, these forms of the disease are rare (Minton and Stanley, 2004). The main route for the infection is fecal–oral, which results from direct contamination or the ingestion of food and water contaminated with the protozoan cyst. The disease affects people who do not live under or do not have access to sanitary conditions. In the United States, the disease is reported mostly among immigrants and those who traveled to developing countries.

Cryptosporidium parvum

Cryptosporidium is an obligate enteric parasite of the phylum Apicomplexa and an important cause of diarrheal disease worldwide. Several species of *Cryptosporidium* are widely distributed among carrier animals and the environment (Egyed et al., 2003). *Cryptosporidium parvum* and *C. hominis* are the main causes of human infection with this protozoal parasite. Cryptosporidiosis has become recognized as one of the most common causes of waterborne disease in the United States, and use of contaminated water easily leads to contamination of produce (Smith and Rose, 1990). Symptoms of the disease include diarrhea, abdominal cramps, and a slight fever. Some cases are without noticeable symptoms. Humans become infected after the ingestion of food or, most commonly, drinking water that is contaminated with the parasite cysts (Meinhardt et al., 1996; Anderson, 1998). Infection can also be contracted by person-to-person transmission and via direct contact with articles contaminated with stool from infected persons, including children. Immunocompromised individuals are at particularly high risk of infection by *Cryptosporidium*.

Cyclospora

Cyclospora cayetanensis was first described in 1979 (see figure 2-4). Symptoms include watery diarrhea with frequent bowel movements, abdominal cramps, nausea, vomiting, muscle aches, and fatigue (Soave et al., 1998). Asymptomatic cases have been documented. Outbreaks of cyclosporiasis have been linked to various types of fresh produce. *Cyclospora* needs days or weeks after being passed in a bowel movement to become infectious. Therefore, it is unlikely that *Cyclospora* is passed directly from one person to another. It is unknown whether animals can be infected and pass infection to people.

Giardia intestinalis

This protozoal parasitic agent causes enteritis characterized by diarrhea, loose or watery stool, and abdominal stomach cramps. The agents live in the intestine of humans and several domestic and wild animals. Giardiasis is one of the most common causes of water-borne diseases in the United States and is worldwide in its distribution. The parasite is passed in the stool of infected persons or animals and may also contaminate foods.

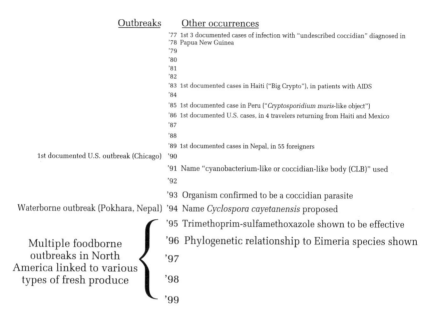

Outbreaks	Other occurrences
	'77 1st 3 documented cases of infection with "undescribed coccidian" diagnosed in
	'78 Papua New Guinea
	'79
	'80
	'81
	'82
	'83 1st documented cases in Haiti ("Big Crypto"), in patients with AIDS
	'84
	'85 1st documented case in Peru (*Cryptosporidium muris*-like object")
	'86 1st documented U.S. cases, in 4 travelers returning from Haiti and Mexico
	'87
	'88
	'89 1st documented cases in Nepal, in 55 foreigners
1st documented U.S. outbreak (Chicago)	'90
	'91 Name "cyanobacterium-like or coccidian-like body (CLB)" used
	'92
	'93 Organism confirmed to be a coccidian parasite
Waterborne outbreak (Pokhara, Nepal)	'94 Name *Cyclospora cayetanensis* proposed
	'95 Trimethoprim-sulfamethoxazole shown to be effective
Multiple foodborne outbreaks in North America linked to various types of fresh produce	'96 Phylogenetic relationship to Eimeria species shown
	'97
	'98
	'99

Figure 2-4. The recognition of previously unknown pathogens in the past three decades includes the discovery of food-borne bacteria, viruses, and protozoa. This figure describes the recent chronology in discoveries regarding *Cyclospora cayetanensis*. Source: Herwaldt (2000). Reprinted by permission, University of Chicago Press, Clinical Infectious Diseases.

Taenia solium

Ingestion of the pork tapeworm eggs can cause a disease called cysticercosis after the tapeworm larvae enter the body and form cysticerci (Schantz and Tsang, 2003). When cysticerci are found in the brain, the condition is called neurocysticercosis. The tapeworm that causes cysticercosis is found worldwide. Tapeworm eggs are passed in the stool of infected person and can contaminate food, water, or soil. Persons who have tapeworm infections can reinfect themselves (autoinfection). Once inside the stomach, the tapeworm egg hatches, penetrates the intestine, travels through the bloodstream, and may develop into cysticerci in the muscles, brain, or eyes, leading to the development of chronic infection with symptoms depending on the location of the infection. Most people with cysticerci in muscles will not have symptoms of infection. However, neurocysticercosis can be characterized with lesions in the brain that can be associated with seizures and headaches as the most common symptoms (Garcia and Brutto, 2005).

Toxoplasma gondii

Toxoplasma gondii are protozoal parasites with a life cycle having three infective stages. Sporozoites are released from oocysts excreted by cats (and other feline species), tachyzoites are forms that multiply in animal cells, and bradyzoites can become encysted in animal tissue. The complexity and variation of these forms create multiple pathways for infection. Human infection follows the ingestion of the oocysts (excreted by cats) or ingestion of meat with the parasite encysted in the tissue. The oocysts can remain in the soil and in water, providing routes of contamination through contact with soil and with produce. Jeffrey et al (2003) . Exposure and serologic evidence of exposure in population studies is common, and infection may be asymptomatic. Pregnant women can pass the infection to their unborn child even if they do not show symptoms. A small percentage of infected newborns have serious eye or brain damage at birth. Immunocompromised individuals are particularly susceptible to toxoplasmosis, and toxoplasmic encephalitis is one of the AIDS-defining opportunistic infections (Eza and Locas, 2006).

Trichinella spiralis

Trichinellosis (trichinosis) may be one of the best-known food-borne pathogens. It is caused by ingestion of raw or undercooked pork and wild game products (bear, wild feline [e.g., a cougar], fox, dog, wolf, horse, seal, or walrus) infected with *Trichinella* cysts, which are the larvae of a species of worm called *Trichinella spiralis*. From 1991 through 1996, an annual average of 38 cases per year were reported (Moorhead et al., 1999). Symptoms of the disease include nausea, diarrhea, vomiting, fatigue, fever, and abdominal discomfort that can last for months at the first stage of the diseases. Additionally, headaches, fevers, chills, cough, eye swelling, aching joints and muscle pains, and itchy skin have also been described.

Laboratory Tests for Parasitic Pathogens

The most common samples submitted to the laboratory for the detection of *Cryptosporidium parvum*, *Cryptosporidium parvum*, *Entamoeba histolytica*, *Giardia lamblia*, and *Toxoplasma gondii* include stool for identification of the specific parasitic stage in intestinal tract, body fluids or tissues for detection of larval stages, and serum samples for the detection of significant titers for parasite-specific antibodies such as in cases of toxoplasmosis.

Viruses

There is increasing awareness of the importance of viral agents in causing food-borne outbreaks and numerous cases of food-borne illness; however, diagnostic testing for viruses is much less developed than that of bacteria, and viral agents are less frequently confirmed by laboratory tests. Viral infections can lead to the inflammation of the stomach and small and large intestines, resulting in vomiting or diarrhea, and gastroenteritis. Viruses that are frequent causes of gastroenteritis include hepatitis A, *Norovirus*, and rotavirus.

Hepatitis A Virus

Hepatitis A virus is a member of the enterovirus group of the Picornaviridae family. The virus is characterized by a single molecule of RNA encased by a small protein shell. The Hepatitis A virus is the most common of the hepatitis viruses, accounting for around 40% of all cases of hepatitis in the United States. According to the CDC, each year in the United States an estimated 143,000 cases of hepatitis A virus infection occur, but only around 30,000 are reported. Infection with hepatitis A causes hepatitis characterized by jaundice, fatigue, abdominal pain, loss of appetite, nausea, diarrhea, and fever. It can result from the direct contact with an infected individual, through fecal–oral route, or by the ingestion of foods and water that are contaminated with the virus from an infected handler. The disease is common among household contacts and sexual contacts of infected persons. Some infected people may suffer from prolonged or relapsing symptoms over a 6–9 month period. The disease can be prevented by the hepatitis A vaccine. A short-term protection against hepatitis A is available from immune globulin. It can be given before and within 2 weeks after coming in contact with hepatitis A.

Caliciviruses

The genus *Norovirus*, family Caliciviridae, is a group of related, single-stranded RNA, nonenveloped viruses that cause acute gastroenteritis in humans. *Norovirus* was recently approved as the official genus name for the group of viruses provisionally described as "Norwalk-like" viruses. This group of viruses has also been referred to as caliciviruses (because of their family name) and as small round structured viruses, or SRSVs (Deneen et al., 2000). Another genus of the calicivirus family that can cause gastroenteritis in humans is *Sapovirus*, formerly described as "Sapporo-like" virus and sometimes referred to as classic or typical calicivirus. Noroviruses are named after the original strain, "Norwalk virus," which caused an outbreak of gastroenteritis in a school in Norwalk, Ohio, in 1968. Currently, there are at least four *Norovirus* genogroups (GI, GII, GIII, and GIV), which in turn are divided into at least 20 genetic clusters. Noroviruses are recognized as the most common cause of acute nonbacterial gastroenteritis in persons older than 5 years and are responsible for more than 90% of nonbacterial gastroenteritis outbreaks (Fankhauser et al., 2002).

Norovirus infection usually manifests as acute-onset vomiting, watery non-bloody diarrhea with abdominal cramps, and nausea. Low-grade fever also occasionally occurs, and vomiting is more common in children. The incubation period for *Norovirus*-associated gastroenteritis in humans is usually between 24 and 48 hours, but cases can occur within 12 hours of exposure. Dehydration is the most common complication, especially among the young and elderly, and may require medical attention. Symptoms usually last 24–60 hours. Recovery is usually complete, and there is no evidence of any serious long-term sequelae. Noroviruses are transmitted primarily through the fecal–oral route, either by consumption of fecally contaminated food or water or by direct person-to-person spread.

Most food-borne outbreaks of *Norovirus* illness are likely to arise though direct contamination of food by a food handler immediately before its consumption. Outbreaks have frequently been associated with consumption of cold foods, including various salads, sandwiches, and bakery products. Liquid items (e.g., salad dressing or cake icing) that allow virus to mix evenly are often implicated as a cause of outbreaks. Food can also be contaminated at its source, and oysters from contaminated waters have been associated with widespread outbreaks of gastroenteritis. Other foods, including raspberries and salads, have been contaminated before widespread distribution and subsequently caused extensive outbreaks. Environmental and fomite contamination may also act as a source of infection.

Noroviruses are highly contagious, and an inoculum of as few as 10 viral particles may be sufficient to infect an individual. During outbreaks of *Norovirus* gastroenteritis, several modes of transmission have been documented, for example, initial food-borne transmission in a restaurant, followed by secondary person-to-person transmission to household contacts. Although presymptomatic viral shedding may occur, shedding usually begins with onset of symptoms and may continue for 2 weeks after recovery. It is unclear to what extent viral shedding more than 72 hours after recovery signifies continued infectivity (Bresee et al., 2002).

Based on the CDC estimates (MMWR 2005), more than 23 million cases of acute gastroenteritis are due to *Norovirus* infection, and it is now thought that at least 50% of all food-borne outbreaks of gastroenteritis can be attributed to noroviruses. Parashar et al., 2001 reported that among the 232 outbreaks of *Norovirus* illness reported to CDC from July 1997 to June 2000, 57% were food-borne, 16% were due to person-to-person spread, and 3% were waterborne; in 23% of outbreaks, the cause of transmission was not determined. In this study, common settings for outbreaks include restaurants and catered meals (36%), nursing homes (23%), schools (13%), and vacation settings or cruise ships (10%).

Rotavirus

Rotaviruses are nonenveloped, double-shelled viruses. The virus is stable in the environment, and transmission can occur through ingestion of contaminated water or food and contact with contaminated surfaces. These viruses are the most common cause of severe diarrhea among children, resulting in the hospitalization of approximately 55,000 children each year in the United States and the death of more than 600,000 children annually worldwide (Rosenfeldt et al., 2005). The primary mode of transmission is fecal–oral. The incubation period for rotavirus disease is approximately 2 days. The disease is characterized by vomiting and watery diarrhea for 3–8 days, and fever and abdominal pain occur frequently. In persons with healthy immune systems, rotavirus gastroenteritis is a self-limited illness, lasting for only a few days. About 1 in 40 children with rotavirus gastroenteritis will require hospitalization for intravenous fluids. Prevention of the disease can be achieved through the prevention of fecal–oral transmission of the virus and the avoidance of foods and water, particularly cold foods, that may be contaminated with the virus (Verboon-Maciolek et al., 2005).

Laboratory Tests for Viral Pathogens

Identification of virus-specific antibodies by immunoassays for IgM, anti-hepatitis A antibody, and certain liver function enzymes (e.g., alanine transferase) will confirm the diagnosis. For food-borne illnesses due to noroviruses, serological findings indicating a high titer (fourfold) to the noroviruses based on acute and convalescent serum samples and negative culture results for potential bacterial agents provide the final diagnosis. Less frequently encountered viral agents, such as rotaviruses, astroviruses, caliciviruses, and adenoviruses, are usually detected by isolation of the virus in early acute stool samples and complemented by immunoassays on sera from affected individuals.

Prions

Prions are infectious protein particles that resist inactivation by heat and digestion and are hypothesized to be the causative agent associated with a group of chronic neurological diseases that follow long latency periods (Enserink, 2005; Colchester and Colchester, 2005). Prions infect human and animal tissue, and consumption of infected tissue may lead to disease. The postmortem appearance of the brain includes large vacuoles in the cortex and cerebellum;

therefore, prion disease is often called spongiform encephalopathy. Prions are hypothesized to be the pathogenic agent causing "mad cow" disease, bovine spongiform encephalopathy (BSE), which was first described in Europe in 1996. Similar spongiform encephalopathies affect several animal species, such as scrapie in sheep, transmissible mink encephalopathy in minks, and chronic wasting disease in muledeer and elks (Xie et al., 2006). Consumption of cattle infected with the BSE prion may cause variant Creutzfeldt-Jakob disease (vCJD) in humans, a rare and fatal degenerative neurologic disease characterized by loss of motor control, dementia, paralysis, wasting, and eventually death (Wilson and Ricketts, 2006).

vCJD is classified as a transmissible spongiform encephalopathy because of the characteristic spongy degeneration of the brain and its ability to be transmitted. vCJD was first described in March 1996 (Collinge et al., 1996). Before the identification of vCJD, CJD was recognized to exist in only three forms: Genetic CJD, which is caused by an inherited abnormal gene, and in most cases the illness is known within the family because of the family history; sporadic cases, which have an unknown cause and occur throughout the world at the rate of about one per million people, and which account for 85–90% of CJD cases; and iatrogenic cases, which result from the accidental transmission of the causative agent via contaminated surgical equipment, from cornea or dura mater transplants, or via administration of human-derived pituitary growth hormones. In January 2002, the U.S. Food and Drug Administration published its new guidance to reduce the theoretical risk of transmission of the agents of CJD and vCJD by blood and blood products (http://www.fda.gov/cber/gdlns/cjdvcjd.htm).

Laboratory Tests for Prions

Year by year, laboratory tests for prion disease are being developed and incorporated into animal health and food safety programs. Two methods for testing slaughtered beef for presence of the BSE prion are the Western blot and immunohistochemistry, both of which are recognized by the World Animal Health Organization as confirmatory tests for BSE. In Western blot, a homogenized sample of central nervous system tissue from cattle or sheep is exposed to the enzyme proteinase K, and the infective prion protein (PrP^{Sc}) can be distinguished from the normal prion protein (PrPc) by protease resistance and molecular size. In the second method, presence of PrP^{Sc} is detected by immunohistochemistry, which results in positive staining in the obex, the appropriate anatomical region for a confirmative diagnosis.

Biological Toxins

Bacterial Toxins

Many food-borne bacteria produce toxins as apart of their virulence factors. The following toxins are well established and are known to be associated with food-borne disease manifestations. *Escherichia coli* enterotoxins cause excess secretion in ligated intestinal segments of rabbits without either histological evidence of intestinal damage or evidence of injury. Some of these toxins may impair electrically neutral NaCl absorption, which also results in net ion secretion. Cytoskeleton-altering toxins such those produced by campylobacters may produce an alteration in cell shape, most often due to rearrangement of F-actin. The toxin may produce limited cell injury but is not lethal to cells and may or may not be associated with evidence of net secretion in *in vivo* or *in vitro* intestinal epithelial cell models of disease. Shiga cytotoxins such those produced by *E. coli* O157:H7, which can cause hemolytic uremia, produce cell or tissue damage, usually culminating in cell death. The toxin may or may not be associated with net secretion in *in vivo* or *in vitro* intestinal epithelial cell models of disease. *Staphylococcus aureus* produces toxin in the food before consumption, which is called "preformed" toxin and is the cause of common staph food poisoning that has a rapid onset within 6 hours of ingestion (Kauffman, 2006).

Clostridium botulinum

Clostridium botulinum, anaerobic bacteria that survive and grow with little or no oxygen, produce botulinum toxin, one of the most potent toxins known in nature and the cause of serious poisoning. *Clostridium botulinum* are usually associated with faulty home canning of vegetables as well as other foods that provide suitable anaerobic growth conditions for the bacterial spores to vegetate and produce the toxins. The toxin affects the nerves and, if untreated, can cause paralysis and respiratory failure. In the United States, an average of 110 cases of food, infant, and wound botulism are reported to the CDC each year (Sobel et al., 2004).

Although many cases of food-borne botulism come from home-canned foods with low acid content, such as asparagus, green beans, beets, and corn, outbreaks of botulism are associated with unusual sources such as chili peppers, tomatoes, and improperly handled baked potatoes wrapped in aluminum foil. In Alaska, the incidence of botulism is among the highest in the world, and all cases of food-borne botulism in Alaska have been associated with eating traditional Alaska Native foods, including "fermented" foods, dried foods, seal oil, and muktuk (skin and a thin pinkish blubber layer immediately underneath the skin) from marine mammals. Botulism toxins are divided into seven types; intoxication with toxin type E is exclusively associated with eating aquatic animals and causes most cases of botulism in Alaska. Botulism death rates among Alaska Natives have declined in the last 20 years, yet incidence has increased. On July 12, 2002, two residents of a Yup'ik village in western Alaska found a carcass of a beached beluga whale that appeared to have died sometime that spring. They collected the tail fluke for consumption, cut it into pieces, and put the pieces in sealable plastic bags. Portions were refrigerated and distributed to family and friends. From July 13 to July 15, a total of 14 persons ate some of the raw muktuk. On July 17, a physician from western Alaska reported three suspected cases of botulism from this village; all patients had eaten the muktuk.

Symptoms of food-borne botulism include double vision and drooping eyelids, slurred speech, dry mouth and difficulty swallowing, and weak muscles. These symptoms begin within 18–36 hours of eating contaminated food but can occur as quickly as 6 hours afterward or can delay for as much as 10 days. When diagnosed early, cases of food-borne botulism can be successfully treated with an antitoxin that blocks the action of the bacterial toxin circulating in the blood. Although antitoxin keeps the disease from becoming worse, recovery still takes many weeks. Severe botulism can cause paralysis of the arms, legs, trunk, and muscles that control breathing, and patients may have to be put on ventilators.

Marine Toxins

Fish and seafood can become contaminated by microorganisms that produce powerful toxins that are not attenuated by cooking. The toxins vary in effect and are specific to each microorganism. For example, scombrotoxic fish poisoning, also known as scombroid or histamine fish poisoning, is caused by bacterial spoilage of tuna, mackerel, bonito, and, rarely, other fish. As bacteria break down fish proteins, by-products such as histamine build up in fish and can cause human disease. Symptoms begin within 2 minutes to 2 hours after eating the fish. The most common symptoms are rash, diarrhea, flushing, sweating, headache, and vomiting. Burning or swelling of the mouth, abdominal pain, or a metallic taste may also occur (Isbister and Kiernan, 2005).

Another type of poisoning, ciguatera poisoning, is caused by eating tropical reef fish contaminated with ciguatoxins produced by microscopic sea plants called dinoflagellates. *Gambierdiscus toxicus* is the dinoflagellate most notably responsible for production of ciguatoxin, although other species have been identified more recently. More than 400 species of fish have been implicated in ciguatera poisoning, starting with herbivores and then climbing up the food chain to the larger carnivorous fish (Lewis and Holmes, 1993). These toxins become progressively concentrated as they move up the food chain from small fish to large fish that eat them, and reach particularly high concentrations in large predatory tropical reef fish. Barracuda are commonly associated with ciguatoxin poisoning, but eating grouper, sea bass, snapper, mullet, and a number of other fish that live in oceans between latitude 35° N and 35° S has caused the disease. Nonspecific symptoms include nausea, vomiting, diarrhea, cramps, excessive sweating, headache, and muscle aches.

Paralytic shellfish poisoning results from the toxin produced by the dinoflagellate *Gymnodinium breve*. These dinoflagellates have a red-brown color and can grow to such numbers that they cause red streaks to appear in the ocean called "red tides." This toxin is known to concentrate within certain shellfish that typically live in the colder coastal waters of the Pacific states and New England, though the syndrome has been reported in Central America. Shellfish that have caused this disease include mussels, cockles, clams, scallops, oysters, crabs, and lobsters. Symptoms begin anywhere from 15 minutes to 10 hours after eating the contaminated shellfish. In cases of severe poisoning, muscle paralysis and respiratory failure occur, and in these cases death may occur in 2–25 hours.

Neurotoxic shellfish poisoning is caused by a third type of dinoflagellate (*Pfiesteria piscicida*) with a toxin that may accumulate in oysters, clams, and mussels from the Gulf of Mexico and the Atlantic coast of the southern states. Symptoms begin 1–3 hours after eating the contaminated shellfish and include numbness, tingling in the mouth, arms and legs, lack of coordination, and gastrointestinal upset (Feldman et al., 2005).

Diagnosis of marine toxin poisoning is generally based on symptoms and a history of recently eating a particular kind of seafood. If suspect leftover fish or shellfish are available, they can be tested for the presence of the toxin more easily. There are few specific treatments for ciguatera poisoning, paralytic shellfish poisoning, or neurotoxic shellfish poisoning. Antihistamines and epinephrine, however, may sometimes be useful in treating the symptoms of scombrotoxic fish poisoning. Long-term consequences have not been associated with paralytic shellfish poisoning, neurotoxic shellfish poisoning, and scombrotoxic fish poisoning.

The most important marine phycotoxins are shellfish toxins and ciguatoxins. Five types of shellfish toxins have been identified:

1. Paralytic shellfish toxins causing paralytic shellfish poisoning (PSP)
2. Diarrhoeic shellfish toxins causing diarrheic shellfish poisoning (DSP)
3. Amnesic shellfish toxins causing amnesic shellfish poisoning (ASP)
4. Neurotoxic shellfish toxins causing neurotoxic shellfish poisoning (NSP)
5. Azaspiracid shellfish toxins causing azaspiracid shellfish poisoning (AZP)

Ciguatoxins cause ciguatera fish poisoning (CFP). PSP, DSP, ASP, NSP, and AZP are caused by human consumption of contaminated shellfish products, whereas CFP is caused by the consumption of subtropical and tropical marine carnivorous fish that have accumulated ciguatera toxins through the marine food chain.

References

Anderson BC. Cryptosporidiosis in bovine and human health. *J Dairy Sci.* 1998; 81(11): 3036–3041.

Aarnisalo K, Autio T, Sjoberg AM, Lunden J, Korkeala H, Suihko ML. Typing of Listeria monocytogenes isolates originating from the food processing industry with automated ribotyping and pulsed-field gel electrophoresis. *J Food Prot.* 2003; 66(2): 249–255.

Blake PA, Merson MH, Weaver RE, Hollis DG, Heublein PC. Disease caused by a marine *Vibrio*. Clinical characteristics and epidemiology. *N Engl J Med.* 1979; 300(1):1–5.

Blaser MJ. Epidemiologic and clinical features of *Campylobacter jejuni* infections. *J Infect Dis.* 1997;176(suppl 2):S103–S105.

Bresee JS, Widdowson M-A, Monroe SS, Glass RI. Food-borne viral gastroenteritis: challenges and opportunities. *Clin Infect Dis.* 2002; 35:748–753.

Centers for Disease Control and Prevention (CDC). Outbreaks of Escherichia coli O157:H7 Infection Associated with Eating Alfalfa Sprouts—Michigan and Virginia, June–July 1997. MMWR August. 1997; *46*(32):741–744

Centers for Disease Control and Prevention (CDC). Multisite outbreak of norovirus associated with a franchise restaurant—Kent County, Michigan, May 2005. MMWR. 2006; *55*(14): 395–397.

Centers for Disease Control and Prevention (CDC). Preliminary FoodNet data on the incidence of infection with pathogens transmitted commonly through food—10 States, United States, 2005. MMWR. 2006; 55(14): 392–395.

Colchester AC, Colchester NT. The origin of bovine spongiform encephalopathy: the human prion disease hypothesis. *Lancet.* 2005; 366(9488):856–861.

Collinge J, Sidle KCL, Meads J, et al. Molecular analysis of prion strain variation and the aetiology of "new variant" CJD. *Nature* 1996; 383:685–690.

Deneen VC, Hunt JM, Paule CR, James RI, Johnson RG, Raymond MJ, et al. The impact of food-borne calicivirus disease: the Minnesota experience. *J Infect Dis.* 2000; 181(suppl 2):S281–S283.

Egyed Z, Sreter T, Szell Z, Varga I. Characterization of *Cryptosporidium* spp.—recent developments and future needs. *Vet Parasitol.* 2003; 111(2–3):103–114.

Ekdahl K, Andersson Y. The epidemiology of travel-associated shigellosis—regional risks, seasonality and serogroups. *J Infect Dis.* 2005; 51(3):222–229.

Enserink M. Spongiform diseases. After the crisis: more questions about prions. *Science.* 2005; 310(5755):1756–1758.

Eza DE, Lucas SB. Fulminant toxoplasmosis causing fatal pneumonitis and myocarditis. HIV Med. 2006; 7(6): 415–420.

Fankhauser RL, Monroe SS, Noel JS, Humphrey CD, Bresee JS, Parashar UD, et al. Epidemiologic and molecular trends of "Norwalk-like viruses" associated with outbreaks of gastroenteritis in the United States. *J Infect Dis.* 2002; 186:1–7.

Feldman KA, Werner SB, Cronan S, Hernandez M, Horvath AR, Lea CS, et al. A large outbreak of scombroid fish poisoning associated with eating escolar fish (Lepidocybium flavobrunneum). *Epidemiol Infect.* 2005; 133(1):29–33.

Fisher IS, Meakins, S. Enter-net participants. Surveillance of enteric pathogens in Europe and beyond: Enter-net annual report for 2004. *Euro Surveill.* 2006; 11(8): E060824.3.

Garcia HH, Del Brutto OH; Cysticercosis Working Group in Peru. Neurocysticercosis: updated concepts about an old disease. *Lancet Neurol.* 2005; 4(10):653–661.

Henrik C & Cheasty.T. The serodiagnosis of human infections with *Yersinia enterocolitica* and *Yersinia pseudotuberculosis.* FEMS Immunology & Medical Microbiology. 2006; 47: 391–397.

Isbister GK, Kiernan MC. Neurotoxic marine poisoning. *Lancet Neurol.* 2005; 4(4):219–228.

Jones JL, Kruszon-Moran D, Wilson M. *Toxoplasma gondii* Infection in the United States, 1999–2000. *Emerg Infect Dis.* 2003;.9(11).

Kauffman NM, Roberts RF. Staphylococcal enterotoxin D production by Staphylococcus aurous FRI100. *J Food Prot.* 2006; 69(6):1448–1451.

Kaper JB. Pathogenic Escherichia coli. *Int J Med Microbiolo.* 2005; 295(6–7): 355–356.

Kist M. The historical background of *Campylobacter* infection: new aspects. In: Pearson AD, editor. *Proceedings of the 3rd International Workshop on Campylobacter Infections*; Ottawa; 1985 Jul 7–10. London: Public Health Laboratory Service; 1985; 23–27.

Lee R, Peppe J, George H.. Pulsed-field gel electrophoresis of genomic digests demonstrate linkages among food, food handlers, and patrons in a food-borne *Salmonella javiana* outbreak in Massachusetts. *J Clin Microbiol.* 1998. 36:284–285.

Lewis RJ, Holmes MJ. Origin and transfer of toxins involved in ciguatera. *Comp Biochem Physiol C.* 1993. 106:615–628.

Meinhardt PL, Casemore DP, Miller KP. Epidemiologic aspects of human cryptosporidiosis and the role of waterborne transmission. *Epidemiol Rev.* 1996; 18(2):118–136.

Minton J, Stanley P. Intra-abdominal infections. *Clin Med.* 2004; 4(6):519–523.

Moorhead A, Grunenwald PE, Dietz VJ, Schantz PM. Trichinellosis in the United States, 1991–1996: declining but not gone. *Am J Trop Med Hygiene* 1999; 60:66–69.

Muller N, von Allmen N. Recent insights into the mucosal reactions associated with *Giardia lamblia* infections. *Int J Parasitol.* 2005; 35(13):1339–1347.

Nachamkin I. Chronic effects of *Campylobacter* infection. *Microbes Infect.* 2002; 4:399–403.

Oliver JD, Kaper JB. *Vibrio* species. In: Doyle MP, Beuchat LR, and Montville TJ, editors. *Food Microbiology. Fundamentals and Frontiers.* American Society of Microbiology Press, Washington, DC; 2001: 263–300.

Parashar U, Quiroz ES, Mounts AW, Monroe SS, Fankhauser RL, Ando T, et al. "Norwalk-like viruses." Public health consequences and outbreak management. *MMWR Recomm Rep.* 2001; 50(RR-9):1–17.

Ribot EM, Fitzgerald C, Kubota K, Swaminathan B, Barrett TJ. Rapid pulsed-field gel electrophoresis protocol for subtyping of *Campylobacter jejuni. J Clin Microbiol.* 2001; 39:1889–1894.

Rosenfeldt V, Vesikari T, Pang XL, Zeng SQ, Tvede M, Paerregaard A. Viral etiology and incidence of acute gastroenteritis in young children attending day-care centers. *Pediatr Infect Dis J.* 2005; 24(11):962–965.

Saeed Am, Lindell KA, Thacker HL. Experimental infection of four strains of commercial laying hens with Salmonella enterica serovar Enteritidis Phage type 8. In *Salmonella enterica Serovar Enteritidis in Humans and Animals* ed. Saeed AM, ed. Ames, IA: Iowa State University Press, 245–254.

Schantz PM, Tsang VC. The US Centers for Disease Control and Prevention (CDC) and research and control of cysticercosis. *Acta Trop.* 2003 87(1):161–163.

Smith HV, Rose JB. Waterborne cryptosporidiosis. *Parasitol Today.* 1990; 6(1):8–12.

Soave R, Herwaldt BL, Relman DA. Cyclospora. *Infect Dis Clin North Am.* 1998; 12(1):1–12.

Sobel J, Tucker N, McLaughlin J, Maslanka S. Food-borne botulism in the United States, 1990–2000. *Emerg Infect Dis.* 2004;10:1606–1611.

Tenover FC, Arbeit RD, Goering RV, Mickelsen PA, Murray BE, Persing DH, et al. Interpreting chromosomal DNA restriction patterns produced by pulsed-field gel electrophoresis: criteria for bacterial strain typing. *J Clin Microbiol.* 1995;33:2233–2239.

Tuttle J, Gomez T, Doyle MP, Wells JG, Zhao T, Tauxe RV, et al. Lessons from a large outbreak of *E. coli* O157:H7 infections: insights into the infectious dose and method of widespread contamination of hamburger patties. *Epidemiol Infect.* 1999; 122(2):185–192.

Verboon-Maciolek MA, Krediet TG, Gerards LJ, Fleer A, van Loon TM. Clinical and epidemiological characteristics of viral infections in a neonatal intensive care unit during 12-year period. *Pediat Iinfect Dis J.* 2005; 24:901–904.

Wallace FM, Call JE, Porto ACS, Cocoma GJ, ERRC Special Projects Team, Luchansky JB. Recovery rate of *Listeria monocytogenes* from commercially prepared frankfurters during extended refrigerated storage. *J Food Prot.* 2003; 66:584–591.

Wilson K, Ricketts MN. A new human genotype prone to variant Creutzfeldt- Jakob disease. *BMJ.* 2006; 332(7551):1164–1165.

Xie Z et al. Chronic wasting disease of elk and deer and Creutzfeldt-Jakob disease: comparative analysis of the scrapie prion protein. *J Biol Chem.* 2006; 281(7):4199–4206.

3

SURVEILLANCE AND DESCRIPTION

Luenda E. Charles and Tamar Lasky

In any effort to apply epidemiologic principles to the study of a group of diseases, the first step entails defining the condition or disease, theoretically and operationally. A simple operational definition of food-borne disease, "a disease of an infectious or toxic nature caused by or thought to be caused by the consumption of food or water," is used by the World Health Organization (WHO) in its surveillance program in Europe (WHO 2003) (see box 3-1). The simplicity is deceptive. Not everyone agrees that waterborne illnesses should be included within food-borne disease; in the United Kingdom, the Food Standards Agency (2002) defines food-borne illness as "caused by the consumption of food contaminated with germs or their toxins." Even if there were complete agreement on the inclusion or exclusion of waterborne illnesses, the key aspect of the definition is that it emphasizes the vehicle or route of transmission, rather than any other factor. If the illness is caused by ingestion of a food containing a biological or chemical agent or physical hazard, the illness is food-borne. If the same exposure and illness is acquired as a result of some other route of transmission (e.g., waterborne, pet-borne, person-to-person contact), the illness is not food-borne. For example, salmonellosis can be a food-borne illness, or it can result from exposure to reptiles such as pet turtles. Shigellosis can be food-borne, but it can also be transmitted by caregivers changing diapers in a daycare setting or through oral–fecal sexual contact.

BOX 3-1 Definitions of Food-Borne Illness

Food Standards Agency (UK)

"Food-borne illness is caused by the consumption of food contaminated with germs or their toxins" (Food Standards Agency, 2002).

WHO Surveillance Program

Food-borne disease: "a disease of an infectious or toxic nature caused by or thought to be caused by the consumption of food or water" (Schmidt and Gervelmeyer, 2003).

CDC Food-Borne Disease Outbreak Surveillance System

Food-borne disease outbreak: "the occurrence of two or more cases of a similar illness resulting from the ingestion of a common food" (Centers for Disease Control, 2000).

Listeriosis can be food-borne, but it can also be transmitted by cross-infection of newborn babies in hospitals. There is no one illness or set of symptoms that can be considered to be 100% food-borne, and there is considerable heterogeneity in the agents that lead to food-borne illness (as described in chapter 2). This presents a challenge to those establishing operational definitions of food-borne illness in outbreak investigations and surveillance systems. When attempting to aggregate data from multiple sources to estimate the burden of food-borne illness, one must consider ways in which an operational definition over- or underestimates the number of cases of illness acquired through food-borne transmission.

Case definition in an outbreak is usually highly specific to the outbreak (see chapter 6). It may begin with the constellation of symptoms reported by the first cases recognized, something as simple as "vomiting with a high fever." If a pathogen is involved and identified, presence of the pathogen in laboratory-confirmed tests may or may not become part of the case definition. This will vary with the feasibility of obtaining specimens and having those specimens tested in the laboratory; those who are ill in outbreaks frequently do not provide the necessary biological specimens. Other case definitions used in outbreaks might require culture-confirmed testing, and if pulsed-field gel electrophoresis (PFGE) testing is done, the cases would need to be of the same PFGE types. Thus, an outbreak definition may vary from a broad, symptomatic description to a highly technical laboratory definition of DNA characteristics. In surveillance systems, case definitions can also vary along the same continuum, from reliance on symptoms (e.g., "Have you had diarrhea in the past 30 days?") to laboratory culture and PFGE typing. However, in contrast with the outbreak situation, where an investigator can identify much of what was eaten by the "cases," surveillance systems generally do not identify the food vehicle leading to illness, nor do they confirm that the case was acquired through food-borne transmission.

There is no readily available characteristic distinguishing a case of food-borne illness from a non-food-borne illness on the basis of laboratory tests or symptoms alone. Instead, surveillance systems measure illnesses from pathogens that are known or thought to be known as predominantly food-borne, hospitalizations for general categories of illness such as gastroenteritis, and symptoms such as diarrhea. Thus, a national surveillance for food-borne illness will count all laboratory-confirmed cases of infections by pathogens such as *Salmonella* or *E. coli* O157:H7 and include cases acquired through several means, for example, water, pets, and personal contact. This becomes a source both of misclassification and overcounting, but the degree of misclassification and overcounting has not been explored scientifically, nor do we have available estimates of the overcount.

Surveillance systems for food-borne illness also have varying sources of undercounting, although these may be somewhat better understood. Surveillance through laboratory-confirmed cases misses the many patients who do not consult their doctor when they are ill with, for example, a bacterial or viral gastrointestinal infection, or whose doctors do not collect biological samples and order laboratory tests. Efforts have been made to estimate the number of cases who do not seek health care and who do not submit specimens for laboratory culture, and we are beginning to have a sense of the volume of cases not showing up in laboratory reporting systems. Laboratories, of course, vary in methodology, techniques, and approaches to testing, introducing other sources of over- or undercounting. The introduction of quick tests with lower sensitivity and specificity leads to other artifactual differences in counts.

Surveillance

As with case definitions in an outbreak, surveillance of cases can monitor symptoms, laboratory tests, and other operational case definitions. The focus in food-borne illness is on infectious diseases and rests on public health surveillance structures, including the notifiable disease and the public health laboratory infrastructure. Increased surveillance for pathogens that are frequently food-borne has developed over the past decade to supplement the infectious disease structures already in place. Additionally, ongoing surveys such as the National Health and Nutrition Examination Survey (NHANES) or the National

Hospital Discharge Survey (NHDS) data can provide annual data on symptoms, hospitalizations, and other measures of food-borne illness.

Surveillance Systems in the United States

National Notifiable Diseases Surveillance System

Congress first authorized collection of morbidity reports in 1878, when the U.S. Marine Hospital Service (forerunner of the Public Health Service) collected reports on cholera, smallpox, plague, and yellow fever. These first reporting systems monitored infectious diseases overseas in order to plan quarantine measures to prevent their spread to the United States. In 1893, Congress gave authority to states and local governments to collect information on these diseases. In 1902 Congress directed the Surgeon General to provide forms for collection of morbidity data.

The key point of this brief historical background is that, to this day, authority to report diseases resides with the states and local governments and not with the federal government. The Council of State and Territorial Epidemiologists (CSTE), with input from the Centers for Disease Control and Prevention (CDC), annually reviews a list of notifiable diseases and recommends changes, additions, or deletions. The states then enact legislation mandating reporting of specific diseases. Although we speak of a National Notifiable Diseases Surveillance System (NNDSS), it is neither national nor a system. The CSTE is a professional organization of 850 members, all of whom work in state, territorial, or local health departments, but it is not, itself, part of any government structure. The federal government (CDC) implements reporting through the National Electronic Telecommunications System for Surveillance and by providing expertise in case definitions, form design, data collection, education, and the like. National reports are issued by the CDC in the *Annual Summary of Notifiable Diseases*, the *Morbidity and Mortality Weekly Report*, and other publications. The NNDSS accepts probable and confirmed cases; a separate system, the Public Health Laboratory Information System, accepts culture-confirmed cases only. In 2005, 61 diseases were considered to be nationally notifiable, including the following diseases that are frequently food-borne: botulism, cryptosporidiosis, cyclosporiasis, enterohemorrhagic *E. coli*, giardiasis, salmonellosis, shigellosis, and trichinosis.

Public Health Laboratory Information System

This refers to a software system for entering, editing, and analyzing data locally on desktop computers and transmitting the data to states and, in turn, to the federal government (Bean et al. 1992). The public health infrasturcture has not uniformly converted to electronic data collection, and the multiple surveillance systems do not necessarily interface with each other. When software is created and installed in specific sites, it shapes the type of data that are collected. In this case, the data consist of laboratory-confirmed cases only (the data are entered in public health laboratories). The system appears to be used to monitor *Salmonella* and *Shigella* only and is also referred to by its two roles, National Salmonella Surveillance System and National Shigella Surveillance system. Algorithms have been developed to detect unusual clusters of *Salmonella* infections.

It should also be noted that managed care facilities, hospitals, and counties have laboratories that then forward laboratory results to the state system with varying levels of completeness and accuracy, and that this changes from year to year as more systems become electronic (Backer et al. 2001; Panackal et al. 2002). The United States does not yet have a comprehensive uniform electronic system for collecting laboratory data at the local and state levels. The implications of this piecemeal approach to data collection with respect to completeness, validity, and bias in the data have not been explored.

FoodNet

In 1996, the Food-Borne Diseases Active Surveillance Network (FoodNet) was created as part of the Emerging Infections Program of the CDC to improve population-based surveillance of infections that are usually food-borne. The CDC and its federal partners, the U.S. Department of Agriculture and the Food and Drug Administration, work with the 10 state health departments in California, Colorado, Connecticut, Georgia, Maryland, Minnesota, New Mexico, New York, Oregon, and Tennessee. From 1996 to 2003, the FoodNet surveillance population increased from five sites with a population of 14.2 million to 10 sites and a population of more than 41 million. The objectives of FoodNet are to determine the burden of and monitor trends in food-borne diseases in the United States and to determine the proportion of food-borne diseases attributable to specific foods.

In 1996, FoodNet began surveillance for laboratory-diagnosed cases of infection with *Campylobacter*, Shiga toxin–producing *E. coli* (STEC) O157, *Listeria monocytogenes*, *Salmonella*, *Shigella*, *Vibrio*, and *Yersinia enterocolitica*. In 1997, FoodNet added surveillance for laboratory-diagnosed cases of *Cryptosporidium parvum* and *Cyclospora cayetanensis*. In 2000, FoodNet began to capture information on non-O157 STEC. By 2005, FoodNet conducted surveillance for infections of seven bacterial pathogens and two parasitic pathogens.

To identify cases, FoodNet personnel contact each clinical laboratory in their surveillance area at regular intervals. It is not clear how the extra contact from CDC staff affects case ascertainment; this might result in a temporary (or continued) artifact of states with FoodNet sites showing higher numbers of food-borne illnesses in both FoodNet surveillance and NNDSS counts, and there might even be an increase in reporting of other diseases, as well. The differences (if any) between FoodNet surveillance and notifiable disease reporting in case ascertainment for infections that are tracked by both systems have not been explored. Cases are counted if they are the first isolation of a pathogen from a person. In calculating the incidence rates, the number of cases of diagnosed infections that FoodNet has identified becomes the numerator, and the population estimate for that year becomes the denominator (see box 3-2).

A pyramid is used to illustrate the relationship between the laboratory-confirmed cases ascertained by surveillance and the many more cases of infection that are not counted because the patient did not seek medical care, the physician did not collect a stool sample, or laboratory tests for the pathogen were not conducted (figure 3-1). To describe the relationship between the laboratory-confirmed cases and the uncounted cases, the CDC conducts periodic surveys of the general population, physicians, and clinical laboratories in the surveillance area.

These surveys estimate the prevalence of diarrhea in the general population, the proportion of persons with diarrhea who seek medical care, the frequency with which physicians request specimens and order laboratory cultures, and the frequency with which laboratories test stool and other specimens for the pathogens under surveillance.

Physicians vary in their probability of requesting a culture for patients who showed symptoms such as bloody stools or diarrhea for more than 3 days, and in their understanding of laboratory testing (Hennessy et al. 2004). Laboratory practices vary regarding pathogens tested and laboratory methods of testing for a given pathogen. Among the laboratories that reported routinely testing for *Salmonella*, *Shigella*, and *Campylobacter* species, only 57% routinely tested for *E. coli* O157:H7, 50% for *Y. enterocolitica*, and 50% for *Vibrio* species (Voetsch et al. 2004). The proportion of laboratories that routinely tested for *E. coli* O157:H7 increased from 59% in 1995 to 68% in 2000; however, the proportion of stool specimens tested decreased from 53% to 46%. Laboratory testing becomes expensive, and as with any screening or diagnostic tool, one wishes to maximize sensitivity and specificity and minimize the cost. Decisions about testing for individual pathogens, and tests used for each pathogen, will vary from laboratory to laboratory. For example, in one study laboratories varied in use of trichrome staining, acid-fast staining, wet mounts, parasitologic examination of tissue and fluid samples, and/or immunoassay for antigen detection to test for parasites (Jones et al. 2004).

PulseNet

Pulsed-field gel electrophoresis allows molecular subtyping of bacterial isolates by comparing the patterns of DNA fragments produced when exposed

---

BOX 3-2 Incidence

FoodNet surveillance measures the incidence of culture-confirmed (laboratory reported) cases of specific pathogens.

Incidence rates require information about the geographic unit (who's in, who's out), the population living in the unit, and the time interval (week, month, quarter, or year).

The yearly incidence rate of, for example, salmonellosis is:

$$\frac{\text{Number of cases of salmonellosis occurring to people living in a geographic unit}}{\text{Number of people living in geographic unit per year}}$$

Because the number is a fraction, it is multiplied by an appropriate order of 10 (1,000, 100,000, or higher) to produce a rate that is expressed in whole numbers: x cases per 100,000 people per year.

---

to specific enzymes. To ensure comparability of results, it might be best to coordinate efforts from a centralized vantage point, but to ensure timeliness of results, it might be best to permit a decentralized approach to molecular subtyping in the United States. PulseNet was established in 1996 by the CDC to optimize comparability and timeliness of subtyping results and availability of data. PulseNet began with 10 laboratories typing a single pathogen (*E. coli* O157:H7). By 2000, 46 state public health laboratories participated, along with the public health laboratories in New York City and Los Angeles County, California, as well as the U.S. Department of Agriculture's Food Safety and Inspection Service Laboratory and the U.S. Food and Drug Administration laboratories in the Center for Food Safety and Applied Nutrition and Center for Veterinary Medicine. Data from PulseNet are used in detecting, investigating, and controlling food-borne outbreaks. For example, an outbreak may be identified in its early stages when PulseNet observes an increase in a specific subtype of a pathogen, or an outbreak can be confirmed as over by showing a substantial decrease in circulation of the outbreak strain in the affected communities. PulseNet can also determine the geographic scope of the outbreak. In 1995, the CDC, with the assistance of the Association of Public Health Laboratories, selected public health laboratories in several states to help transfer standardized PFGE typing and pattern analysis technology to the area laboratories. For each bacterial pathogen, the PFGE pattern is associated with a pattern database and a database of epidemiologic and clinical information for isolates.

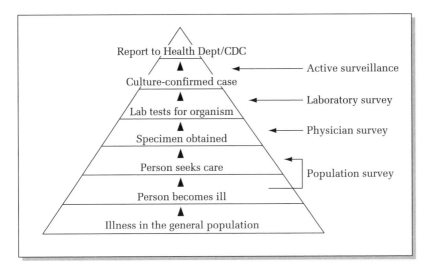

Figure 3-1. The "burden of illness pyramid" used by FoodNet to assess the burden of food-borne disease in the United States. Source: Hardnett et al. (2004).

International Surveillance Systems

The globalization of the food supply and the frequency of international travel create an imperative to monitor food-borne illness throughout the world. Nations develop their own surveillance systems as part of their public health infrastructure. These data are used to protect the health of each country's citizens and also allow countries to coordinate efforts to identify and control food-borne outbreaks when an outbreak threatens to spread beyond a nation's borders. With travel, and constant import and export of food, food-borne illnesses can travel rapidly; prompt information can help limit the spread of illness. The WHO Surveillance Programme for Control of Foodborne Infections and Intoxications in Europe coordinates information from European countries and centralizes reports from individual countries (Schmidt and Gervelmeyer 2003). The program, founded in 1980, now includes 51 of the 52 members of the WHO European region. Much of their work focuses on harmonization of definitions and standardization of methodologies, and they also publish annual reports for each participating country. In addition to information about the official notification system and reported cases in each country, they describe epidemiologically investigated outbreaks.

A report is published for each individual country. Of course, different foods appear in the lists of each country, reflecting the underlying differences in eating habits, as well as potential differential risks in different countries. Quarterly and monthly publications serve to share information across countries and include information from the United States, Canada, and other non-European countries. The Public Health Agency of Canada produces an annual surveillance report describing *Salmonella, Campylobacter*, and pathogenic *E. coli* and *Shigella*. The Communicable Disease Network Australia has modeled its surveillance system, OzNet, on the United States' FoodNet. SIRVETA (Sistema de Informacion para la Vigilancia de las Enfermedades Transmitidas por Alimentos) is the system for Central and South American statistics, and a surveillance system is maintained in Japan by the National Institute of Infectious Disease.

Enter-Net

Enter-Net is an international network for the surveillance of human gastrointestinal infections (Fisher, 1999). The goals of the Enter-Net project are to improve understanding of the extent and evolution of antimicrobial resistance in *Salmonella* isolates and of the distribution of verocytotoxin–producing *E. coli* (VTEC) O157 infections in the European Union. The network monitors salmonellosis and VTEC O157, and their antimicrobial resistance. It is funded by the European Commission and represents a continuation of the Salm-Net surveillance network (1994–1997), which concentrated on harmonization of *Salmonella* phage typing and the establishment of a regularly updated international *Salmonella* database. Originally, Enter-Net involved all 15 countries of the European Union, plus Switzerland and Norway. Salm-Net showed, through the recognition of outbreaks and investigation, that the timely exchange of information between experts in different European Union countries could lead to effective public health action in Europe and beyond. Enter-Net is continuing to extend these benefits to the prevention of *E. coli* O157 infections for each country. The participants in Enter-Net comprise the microbiologist in charge of the national reference laboratory and the epidemiologist responsible for national surveillance.

Descriptive Epidemiology

Variables Associated with Occurrence of Food-Borne Illness— Determinants, Risk Factors, or Other Exposures

In both the acute outbreak and the aggregate of all cases of food-borne illness, descriptive epidemiology is the first step in identifying causal patterns and factors contributing to the occurrence of food-borne illness. Collection of descriptive data in an outbreak is described in chapter 6. This chapter discusses the variables of person, place, and time as they relate to the overall patterns of food-borne illness. This is analogous to the approach used in chronic disease epidemiology where risk factors are identified and studied to help target education, prevention, and intervention.

Person: Age, Sex, Race/Ethnicity, Immune Status

Incidence and severity of infectious food-borne illnesses may vary by age, as they do for most infectious diseases, with young children having little or no immunity to pathogens they have not yet encountered and older people having lost their immunity or being less able to recover from contracted illness. In addition to biological changes over the lifespan (e.g., development of the digestive and immune systems), diet and behavior change dramatically. The incidence of *Salmonella*, the most common cause of food-borne infections, is highest in children younger than 12 months; the rate then declines in children 1–10 years of age and declines further in persons 11–20, after which it remains fairly constant in all other age groups (figure 3–2; Centers for Disease Control and Prevention 2005). The incidences of *Shigella* and *E. coli* O157:H7 follow a different pattern, increasing after the first year of life, declining after age 10, and then leveling off in remaining decades. The incidences of *Listeria* and *Vibrio* infections both appear to show increases with age (older than 40 for *Vibrio*, and older than 60 for *Listeria*). The incidence of *Listeria* is also higher in children younger than 12 months and so combines features of different age distributions. The causes and interpretations of different patterns by age for different pathogens have not been explored.

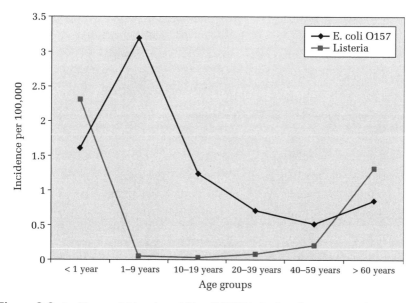

Figure 3-2. Incidence of *Listeria* and *E. coli* O157 infections by age group in FoodNet sites, 2003. Graph developed from data from Centers for Disease Control and Prevention (2005).

A more detailed analysis of the role of age in children younger than 5 shows unique incidence patterns over the first five years of life for six pathogens (Koehler et al. 2006). In this age group, the relationship between age and incidence is more complex than previously thought (figure 3-3). Infections with *E. coli* O157 appear to increase slightly after the first year of life and taper off toward the end of the first five years, while *Shigella* infections peak sharply after age 2 and then decline sharply. Infections from other pathogens appear to be highest in the first year of life and then decline through age 5. These patterns may provide clues about routes of transmission; the peak of *Shigella* infections at age 3 might reflect the contribution of infections acquired through contact with other children. Foods change over the first five years of life (hamburgers are not eaten very much by most infants younger than 12 months, which may explain the lower *E. coli* O157 rates in that age group), and children's contact with dirt, the floor, pets, and other exposures also changes over the first five years of life.

Men and women spend different amounts of time preparing food, may have different habits when preparing food, and may eat in different environments (at a daycare center or camping out on a deer hunt, at restaurants, and many other contexts). It would be reasonable to expect different patterns of illness between the sexes, but it is difficult to predict how these behaviors influence

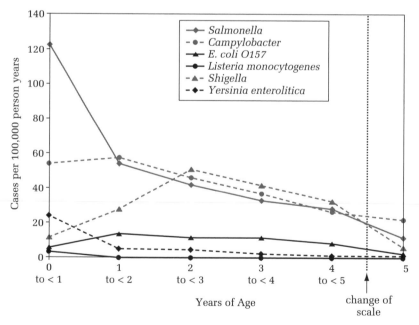

Figure 3-3. Incidence of six pathogens by age, for children younger than 5. Source: Koehler et al. (2006), used with permission.

overall risk levels. FoodNet surveillance data provide information about the distribution of cases of food-borne illness by sex (Centers for Disease Control and Prevention 2003a). From these data, the relative risk can be calculated (table 3-1). An additional effort to obtain denominator data by sex would permit the reader to calculate the 95% confidence intervals around the relative risk (because of the large population under surveillance, 95% confidence intervals would be narrow and might not overlap 1, except for where the point estimate is 1). For six of the pathogens listed in table 3-1, the relative risk is very close to 1. Even if the 95% confidence intervals do not overlap 1, the magnitude of the increase or decrease associated with being male or female is small. This indicates that the risks of infection with *Cyclospora, E. coli* O157, *Listeria, Salmonella, Shigella,* and *Yersinia* are similar for males and females. The risk of campylobacteriosis appears to be 30% higher in males than females, and the risks of infection with *Cryptosporidium* and with *Vibrio* are 60% and 50% higher in males than females. The reasons for these differences have not been explored. The increased exposure in preparing foods at home (traditionally a female role) might increase the risk of exposure to raw and uncooked products and, in turn, to pathogens. This increased exposure might be counterbalanced against the increased risk of eating outside the home (traditionally more males would eat outside the home) and result in fewer differences between males and females. Again, these hypotheses have yet to be explored.

Race and ethnicity may serve as markers for other variables that are risk factors for food-borne illness. Diet and food preparation habits are strongly associated with culture, ethnicity, and race, which are also associated with

TABLE 3-1   Incidence of bacterial and parasitic infections by sex (FoodNet sites, 2003), and relative risk associated with sex (incidence in males/incidence in females)

Infection	Incidence (per 100,000)		Relative Risk
	Male	Female	
Campylobacter	14.07	11.14	1.3
Cryptosporidium	1.43	0.87	1.6
Cyclospora	0.03	0.04	0.8
E. coli O157	0.99	1.13	0.9
Listeria	0.3	0.36	0.8
Salmonella	13.77	14.95	0.9
Shigella	7.43	7.06	1.1
Vibrio	0.32	0.21	1.5
Yersinia	0.39	0.39	1.0

Source: Centers for Disease Control and Prevention (2003a).

education, lifestyle, income, and many other variables related to food choices. Thus, we find Alaskan natives at high risk for botulism infection because of their high consumption of fermented beaver tails, a native food eaten only in Alaska. Food preparation practices also vary with race and ethnicity, so home preparation during the Christmas season of chitterlings (pork intestines) in African-American families in the southern United States is associated with a high incidence of yersiniosis (Ray et al. 2004; Lee et al. 1991). A preference for rare pork has been associated with outbreaks of trichinosis in Asian-American populations, and home-prepared cheeses have been associated with outbreaks of listeriosis and salmonellolis among some Hispanic groups (Linnan et al. 1988; McAuley et al. 1992; Bell et al. 1999). Race and ethnicity are often correlated with education and income, which in turn are associated with knowledge about food safety and inversely related to dependence on purchase of foods past due dates, reliance on soup kitchens, and other practices that may lead to a higher risk of food-borne illness. These hypotheses have not been examined, but it seems intuitive that individuals with fewer economic options might take greater risks with respect to food safety.

A first step in understanding racial and ethnic disparities in the occurrence of food-borne illness is to collect data about race and ethnicity. Although FoodNet surveillance collects data on race and ethnicity, it relies on state reporting systems that vary in the completeness with which they report race and ethnicity, and the level of completeness limits the validity of inferences drawn from the data. The CDC has not published information regarding data quality of their data bases (e.g., information about completeness of data collection for the variables of race and ethnicity), but several publications reporting FoodNet results include discussions of the incomplete coverage of data for race and ethnicity. In the summary of giardiasis surveillance from 1998–2002, data on race were missing for 39.2–46.8% of cases, and data on ethnicity were missing for 49.5–54.5% of cases (Hlavsa et al. 2005). The authors did not analyze the incidence by race or ethnicity, stating that "because data on race and ethnicity are incomplete, conclusions cannot be made about the differences noted in the epidemiology of giardiasis among members of different racial populations and between Hispanics and non-Hispanics" (Hlavsa et al., p. 13).

In the study of *Yersinia enterocolitica*, race and ethnicity were available for 433 of the 527 cases (82%) (Ray et al. 2004). The authors analyzed the data by assuming the same racial and ethnic distribution for cases with race and ethnicity missing as was observed in the cases with race and ethnicity reported. Are cases with missing data similar in racial and ethnic makeup to cases with information available? It would depend on the factors associated with completeness of data, and this has yet to be explored. Reporting of race and ethnicity may vary by state, county, laboratory, or other factors. It is not clear that the distribution of race and ethnicity would be the same in cases with missing data compared to cases with reported data. With respect to the discussion of data quality in chapter 8, bias can be introduced if some racial or ethnic groups are more or less likely to have their race and ethnicity reported (e.g., if an ethnic or racial group lives in a jurisdiction with better or worse reporting). Until reporting of race and ethnicity is more complete, it is difficult to use FoodNet data to assess racial and ethnic disparities in food-borne illness, or to understand reasons for the differences. It would also be questionable to rely on racial and ethnic data from a different country and expect it to explain racial and ethnic patterns of food-borne illness in the United States. At present, the FoodNet data do not permit epidemiologists to fully analyze the issues related to race, ethnicity, and food-borne illness in the United States.

Persons whose immune systems are compromised are at increased risk for food-borne infections and often suffer severe consequences of infection. Pregnant women fall in this group, as do persons with AIDS and persons on immuno-suppressive therapy (e.g., cancer and transplant patients). Because immune status is not available in administrative and surveillance data bases, supplementary studies and analyses are needed to estimate the risk to these sub-populations, and special efforts are needed to target appropriate educational information. Food-borne infections affect these populations in two ways: by increasing the risk of infection and/or by increasing the severity of illness or sequelae once infection occurs. The increased risk of infection is well illustrated by the rates observed in persons already infected with HIV. By 1987, the increased risk of cryptosporidiosis and toxoplasmic encephalopathy in HIV patients was documented and included in the case definition for AIDS (Centers for Disease Control and Prevention 1987; Selik et al. 1987). Since that time, increased risk for campylobacteriosis has been described (Molina et al. 1995). Unfortunately, these food-borne infections may become chronic, or progress, as in the case of toxoplasmosis, to infect the brain, causing dementia (Sacktor et al. 2001). A similar increase in severity and progression has been described in patients with cancer (Israelski and Remington 1993).

It has not been documented whether pregnant women have an increased risk of infection, but the consequences of infection during pregnancy may be more severe, leading to miscarriage, congenital transmission to the fetus, and sequelae of infection in the newborn child. Listeriosis affects pregnant women more seriously than most other food-borne diseases (Smith 1999; Kendall et al. 2003). The disease can result in preterm labor, spontaneous abortion, stillbirth, early-onset infection in the newborn, or birth of a severely ill infant, because this organism is capable of crossing the placenta and directly affecting the fetus. Newborn babies may also acquire infection after birth from the mother or from other infected infants.

Place: Geography

Humidity, ambient temperature, population density, water supply, wild and domestic animal reservoirs, microbiological fauna, and other factors may lead to differences in rates of food-borne illness by geographic area, although the interrelationship between these factors has not been fully described. Michel et al. (1999) studied the geographic distribution of 3,001 cases of *E. coli* O157:H7 infection in Ontario, Canada, and found that areas with a high density of livestock were the areas with highest incidences of infections. They suggest that the presence of cattle leads to contamination of well water or locally produced food products and, in turn, human infections. Curriero et al. (2001) analyzed the relationship between waterborne disease outbreaks and precipitation events above the 90th and 80th percentiles for the watershed area where the outbreaks occurred and found that surface water contamination and outbreaks in the same month were strongly associated. Although both these analyses address waterborne cases and outbreaks, waterborne cases are included in many surveillance systems for food-borne diseases and thus contribute to patterns of variation.

In addition to geographic variation, political boundaries create administrative structures that vary in their ability to ascertain and identify cases of food-borne illnesses, and socioeconomic conditions vary with geography and political boundaries, resulting in variation in eating habits, lifestyle, and access to health care. People vary in their willingness to consult a physician, physicians vary in their use of diagnostic procedures, and states vary in their reporting systems. The sum of these numerous sources of variation result in extreme variations in incidence of specific food-borne infections by state and other geographic units without a recognizable pattern. For example, in 2004, the highest and lowest rates of infection with *Salmonella* were found in Georgia and Oregon, respectively (table 3-2). The highest and lowest rates of infection with *Campylobacter* were found in California and Georgia, and the highest and lowest rates of infection with *Shigella* were found in Georgia and Minnesota. There does not seem to be a state with consistently higher or lower infections for all pathogens. In addition to variation in incidence rates, the magnitude of variation across FoodNet sites is different for each pathogen: in 2004, it was about twofold for *Salmonella* infections but approximately fivefold for *Campylobacter* infections and eight- to ninefold for *Shigella* infections.

Time: Annual Trends and Seasonality

One of the most critical questions that can be asked in public health is whether the incidence of illness is going up or down. Consumers, public health officials, and many others want to know if the danger of food-borne illness is increasing, or if public health interventions are successful in decreasing the occurrence of

TABLE 3-2   Incidence Rates for *Campylobacter, Salmonella, Yersinia,*
and *Shigella* infections in California, Georgia, Minnesota, Oregon, and
New York

	State				
Infection	California	Georgia	Minnesota	Oregon	New York
Campylobacter	28.6	6.6	17.7	18	11.4
Salmonella	14.8	21.9	12.7	10.4	10.5
Yersinia	7.8	4.7	4.3	4.2	2.3
Shigella	7	7.4	1.3	2.2	5

illness. The answers to these questions sometimes depend on how far back in time one looks. If one compares the incidence of most food-borne infections in 2000 to that in 1900, there has been a steep decline. Food-borne infections such as typhoid fever, scarlet fever, and botulism were common in the early 1900s. With improved sanitation, the invention of refrigerators with freezer compartments and common use in homes, and the invention of pasteurization for milk, the incidence of food-borne disease started to decrease.

If one wishes to measure the change in incidence in recent years in the United States, FoodNet data provide incidence rates for selected geographic areas beginning in 1996. Trends can be assessed for all reported cases of food-borne disease or can be assessed after removing all reported cases involved in outbreaks and using data only on sporadic disease cases. The number of sites and the population under surveillance have doubled since FoodNet began in 1996. To account for the increased population and variation in the incidence among sites, FoodNet used a log-linear Poisson regression model to estimate the effect of time on the incidence of the various pathogens, treating time (i.e., calendar year) as a categorical variable. Using 1996 as the reference year, the relative change in incidence rates during 1996–2001 was estimated and the 95% confidence intervals calculated (Centers for Disease Control and Prevention 2003b). In addition to controlling for site-to-site variation and the increasing population, the Poisson regression model incorporates all of the data and will eventually include demographic characteristics such as race, sex, and age (Hardnett et al. 2004).

FoodNet assumes that the proportion at each step of the FoodNet surveillance pyramid remains constant over time. In the United States, the 2003 incidence of infection for most pathogens was lower than the average annual incidence for 1996–1998 (Centers for Disease Control and Prevention 2004). During 1996–2003, the estimated incidence of several infections declined significantly. The estimated incidence of *Yersinia, E. coli* O157, *Campylobacter,* and *Salmonella* infections decreased 49%, 42%, 28%, and 17%, respectively, but the estimated incidence of *Shigella* and *Listeria* infections did not change significantly during that period. The decrease in *E. coli* O157 infections occurred primarily during 2002–2003. The incidence of *Vibrio* infections increased 116%, and *Listeria* did not continue to decline in 2003, as observed during the preceding four years.

Season of the year is another variable associated with multiple variables that may increase or decrease the risk of food-borne illness, including temperature, humidity, eating habits, and lifestyle habits. Again, the interrelationships between these and other related variables have not been fully described. Seasonal temperature and humidity are clearly related to microbial growth rates but also affect temperature in homes, storage temperature for foods and packed lunches, and temperature of foods eaten outdoors. Behaviors and lifestyle also change with the season; people eat differently in warm and cold weathers, and seasonal holidays are associated with different foods throughout the year. While the incidence of many bacterial infections increases in the summer months because of warmer temperatures and increased microbial growth, yersiniosis infections increase in the fall and winter because the main vehicle of transmission, pig intestines, is handled and prepared in the fall and winter, following the traditional pattern of slaughtering hogs in the fall. The custom of eating pork chitterlings in the fall and winter remains even in homes that do not slaughter their own hogs but purchase pork intestine from a butcher or supermarket.

The two peak seasons for common source outbreaks of *Campylobacter* are May and October; there are fewer outbreaks during the summer (Centers for Disease Control and Prevention 2002). In contrast, the numbers of *Campylobacter* isolates of sporadic illnesses reported to the CDC are highest in the summer months. In 2000, the CDC reported 45% of *E. coli* O157 isolates, 37% of *Campylobacter* isolates, and 37% of *Shigella* isolates during the period of June through August. The increase in bacterial disease incidence during summer probably occurs because the warmer temperature allows bacterial pathogens to grow more rapidly in food (Gerber et al. 2002). The water temperature is an important factor for viability and reproducibility of *Vibrio parahemolyticus* and *V. vulnificus* (Shapiro et al. 1998; Daniels et al. 2000), and as expected, *Vibrio* infection in humans occurs mostly in the warmer months of the year.

Variables Associated with Occurrence of Food-Borne Illness— Outcomes and Sequelae

Number of Cases, Hospitalizations, and Deaths

A positive laboratory culture is one outcome of infection, but the impact of disease is also measured by the effect on the public well-being—as days missed from work, dollars spent on health care, visits to health care providers, hospitalizations, and deaths. Using FoodNet surveillance data and information from national health surveys, periodic attempts have been made to go beyond counts of culture-confirmed cases and to estimate the underlying number of cases of food-borne illness, hospitalizations for food-borne illness, and deaths from food-borne illnesses.

The most comprehensive effort to estimate the burden of illness in the United States was the analysis by Mead et al. (1999). Estimates of the total number of cases (reported or nonreported) were based on assumptions about the level of underreporting; the authors assumed 38 underreporting cases of salmonellosis for every reported case but only two cases of unreported listeriosis for every reported cases. They varied the assumptions based on the severity of symptoms, assuming that severe cases were more likely to receive medical attention. Underreporting would decrease with severity of symptoms, and thus a lower multiplier was used for pathogens with generally more severe symptoms. They then developed assumptions for the percentages of cases that were food-borne. They assumed that 100% of all *Clostridium botulinum* cases and 20% of *Shigella* cases were food-borne. The assumptions might bear further review, particularly for the pathogens where no percentage is specified. For *Campylobacter* and *Salmonella*, the authors provided language to the effect that while other forms of transmission are known, the diseases are primarily acquired through food-borne transmission. These assumptions can be readily studied through epidemiologic methods, for example, by studying random samples of cases to estimate the proportions acquired through specific routes of transmission. It is also possible to estimate the variation or uncertainty around the estimates, something that is essential for risk assessment and policy analysis (see chapters 9 and 13).

To estimate the number of hospitalizations for food-borne illnesses, Mead et al. (1999) applied hospitalization rates from reported outbreaks or other published studies to the estimates of the number of cases. They then compared these estimates to National Hospital Discharge Survey data to infer the number of hospitalizations for illnesses where the pathogen was known and where etiology was unknown. Similar comparison to mortality data resulted in estimates of deaths because of food-borne illness. To estimate food-related illnesses and deaths from unknown pathogens, the authors used symptom-based data to estimate the total number of acute gastrointestinal illnesses and then subtracted from this total the number of cases accounted for by known pathogens. This difference represented the illness due to acute gastroenteritis of unknown etiology. After summing illnesses attributable to food-borne gastroenteritis caused by known and unknown pathogens, they arrived at an estimate of 76 million illnesses, 318,574 hospitalizations, and 4,316 deaths. Adding to these figures the nongastrointestinal illness caused by *Listeria*, *Toxoplasma*, and hepatitis A virus, they obtained a final national estimate of 76 million illnesses, 323,914 hospitalizations, and 5,194 deaths each year (figure 3-4).

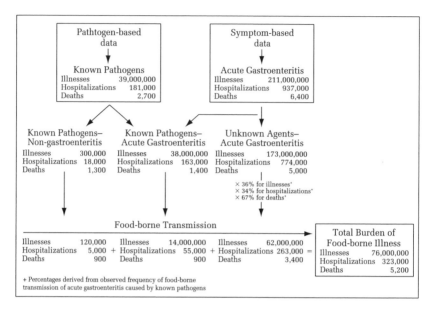

Figure 3-4. Estimated frequency of food-borne illness and death in the United States. +Percentages derived from observed frequency of food-borne transmission of acute gastroenteritis caused by known pathogens. Source: Mead et al. (1999).

Issues in defining cases of food-borne illness are discussed above. In many respects, it is even more difficult to identify deaths caused by food-borne illness. Deaths are assigned causes of death when death certificates are completed (see table 3-3). Some causes of death are food-borne illnesses only, for example, A05, "Other bacterial food-borne intoxications" (poisonings). In most cases, cause of death describes the illness, whether food-borne or not, for example, shigellosis (A03) or acute hepatitis A (B15). One cannot tell whether the illness was food-borne by the infection listed as the cause of death. When the pathogen has not been identified, the cause of death may be listed as "gastroenteritis of unknown etiology," but again, there is no indication whether the gastroenteritis was food-borne or otherwise acquired. A further complication is that death certificates contain space for the immediate cause of death, cause leading to immediate cause, next antecedent cause of death, and the underlying cause of death. For a healthy person who becomes ill with a food-borne illness, the illness would be the immediate cause of death as well as the underlying cause of death, but for a person with AIDS, the food-borne illness might be the immediate cause of death, and AIDS would be the underlying cause of death. Since national statistics are summarized by underlying cause of death, deaths precipitated by food-borne infections would not be counted in national summaries. Conversely, the number of persons with AIDS who die of opportunistic infections as the immediate cause of death can greatly inflate estimates of overall mortality rates for specific infections, as explored in the analyses of Selik et al. (1997), who calculated the proportion of deaths from specific infections with HIV as the underlying cause of death. They found, for example, that 94% of deaths from toxoplasmosis were in people with HIV as the underlying cause of death, and similarly, that 95% of deaths from cryptosporidiosis were in people with HIV as the underlying cause of death. While the immune-incompetent population may die from these infections, the mortality rate for the general population is much smaller than that of the population of people living with AIDS, given infection with the same pathogens. Because of the large contribution of AIDS to mortality from infections, mortality rates may need to be adjusted downward when developing risk estimates for the general population.

Another approach to estimating deaths from food-borne illness would be to identify laboratory-confirmed infections and link the data to death certificates to find out if those with infections die in a given interval following the

TABLE 3-3   International Classification of Diseases, version 10 (ICD-10): Codes for certain infectious and parasitic diseases

(A00–A09) Intestinal infectious diseases
- (A00) Cholera
- (A01) Typhoid and paratyphoid fevers
  - (A01.0) Typhoid fever
- (A02) Other Salmonella infections
- (A03) Shigellosis
- (A04) Other bacterial intestinal infections
  - (A04.0) Enteropathogenic E. coli infection
  - (A04.5) Campylobacter enteritis
  - (A04.6) Enteritis due to Yersinia enterocolitica
  - (A04.7) Enterocolitis due to Clostridium difficile
- (A05) Other bacterial food-borne intoxications
  - (A05.0) Food-borne staphylococcal intoxication
  - (A05.1) Botulism
  - (A05.2) Food-borne Clostridium perfringens (Clostridium welchii) intoxication
- (A06) Amebiasis
- (A07) Other protozoal intestinal disease
  - (A07.0) Balantidiasis
  - (A07.1) Giardiasis (lambliasis)
  - (A07.2) Cryptosporidiosis
  - (A07.3) Isosporiasis
- (A08) Viral and other specified intestinal infections
  - (A08.0) Rotaviral enteritis
- (A09) Diarrhea and gastroenteritis of presumed infectious origin

(B15–B19) Viral hepatitis
- (B15) Acute hepatitis A

positive culture. In such an exercise, one uses the death certificate to confirm vital status, but not necessarily to supply cause of death. The FoodNet system attempts to link its cases to death certificate data to determine fatality rates; again, these are a subset of cases because so many people do not obtain medical care or submit stool specimens. In 2003, FoodNet surveillance reported 83 deaths from laboratory-confirmed infections of food-borne illnesses, as follows: *Salmonella*, 34; *Listeria*, 22; *Campylobacter*, 9; *Vibrio*, 7; *E. coli* O157, 4; *Cryptosporidium*, 3; *Shigella*, 2; and *Yersinia*, 2 (Centers for Disease Control and Prevention 2003a). The cachement population was 41,850,620; the mortality rate from all the identified deaths assumed to be from the food-borne infections followed by FoodNet was 1.98 per million per year.

Sequelae

The consequences of food-borne illness range from mild discomfort and a few days' absence from school or work to hospitalization and death, as mentioned above. Some infections can be followed by distinct medical conditions that are often worse than the infection itself.

Guillain-Barré syndrome (GBS) is a rare paralysis that follows some vaccines and some viral and bacterial infections. Infection with *Campylobacter jejuni* is thought to increase the risk from 1/100,000 to 1/1,000 (MacCarthy and Giesecke 2001). While this is still a rare event, GBS may require months of hospitalization and rehabilitative care and is thus an extremely costly sequela of infection with *C. jejuni*.

Infection of the mother during pregnancy may infect the fetus, resulting in neonates with congenitally acquired disease. For example, mothers infected by the parasite *Toxoplasma gondii* can give birth to infants with congenital toxoplasmosis, and this condition can in turn lead to blindness in the infant. The blindness of the infant is a sequela far more severe than the mother's illness in most cases. Similarly, infection with *Listeria* during pregnancy is thought to be associated with miscarriages, for many women a more severe event than the illness itself.

Hemolytic uremic syndrome (HUS) can occur after an infection of the digestive system by *E. coli* bacterium, whether food-borne or, for example, contracted after swimming in water contaminated with feces. The gastroenteritis caused by *E. coli* is generally confined to vomiting, stomach cramps, and bloody diarrhea, but after 2 or 3 days HUS may develop when the bacteria lodged in the digestive system make toxins that enter the bloodstream and start to destroy red blood cells. Signs and symptoms of HUS may not become apparent until a week later and may include small, unexplained bruises or bleeding from the nose or mouth that may occur because the toxins also destroy the platelets, cells that normally help the blood to clot. The greatest danger is kidney failure—urine formation slows because the damaged red blood cells clog the tiny blood vessels in the kidneys, and the body's inability to rid itself of excess fluid and wastes may lead to high blood pressure or swelling.

E. coli O157:H7 is the predominant pathogen and serotype that is responsible for this illness, but other serotypes of *E. coli* can also cause HUS, which develops in approximately 15% of patients younger than 10 years with a diagnosed *E. coli* O157:H7 infection. While the majority of patients recover from this acute illness, chronic sequelae such as renal problems (most common), diabetes mellitus, neurological disorders, and hypertension may affect some patients. Estimates of the death rate vary; one case series in Canada reported four deaths in a series of 104 children with postdiarrhea HUS (Robson et al. 1991). Because of its severity, the CDC began active surveillance for pediatric HUS cases in 1997 through a network of pediatric nephrologists and infection control practitioners.

Although surveillance of disease and description of co-variates are considered by many to be simple epidemiologic activities, the case-definition for food-borne illness presents particular challenges, as it depends on unverified assumptions about the route of transmission of a number of pathogens, and also depends on the willingness of individuals to seek medical care (and for their physician to collect specimens and order laboratory tests) for food-borne illness. The databases that provide information about laboratory test results contain limited information about co-variates such as race/ethnicity, co-morbidities, and pregnancy status, and no information about exposures. Surveillance for food-borne illness has made great progress in the past decade, however the work in fully describing the epidemiology of food-borne illness has just begun.

Note: The findings and conclusions in this chapter are those of the authors and do not necessarily represent the views of the National Institute for Occupational Safety and Health.

References

Backer, H. D., S. R. Bissell, et al. (2001). "Disease reporting from an automated laboratory-based reporting system to a state health department via local county health departments." *Public Health Rep* 116(3): 257–265.

Bean, N. H., S. M. Martin, et al. (1992). "PHLIS: an electronic system for reporting public health data from remote sites." *Am J Public Health* 82(9): 11273–1276.

Bell, R. A., V. N. Hillers, et al. (1999). "The Abuela Project: safe cheese workshops to reduce the incidence of *Salmonella* Typhimurium from consumption of raw-milk fresh cheese." *Am J Public Health* 89(9): 1421–1424.

Centers for Disease Control and Prevention. (1987). "Revision of the CDC surveillance case definition for acquired immunodeficiency syndrome. Council of State and Territorial

Epidemiologists; AIDS Program, Center for Infectious Diseases." *MMWR Morb Mortal Wkly Rep* 36(suppl 1): 1S–15S.

Centers for disease Control and Prevention (2000). "Surveillance for foodborne Disease Outbreaks—United States, 1993–1997." *MMWR* 49(SS01):1–51.

Centers for Disease Control and Prevention. (2002). FoodNet Annual Report 2002. Atlanta: U.S. Department of Health and Human Services.

Centers for Disease Control and Prevention. (2003a). FoodNet Annual Report 2003. Atlanta: U.S. Department of Health and Human Services.

Centers for Disease Control and Prevention. (2003b). "Preliminary FoodNet data on the incidence of foodborne illnesses—selected sites, United States, 2002." *MMWR Morb Mortal Wkly Rep* 52(15): 340–343.

Centers for Disease Control and Prevention. (2004). "Preliminary FoodNet data on the incidence of infection with pathogens transmitted commonly through food—selected sites, United States, 2003." *MMWR Morb Mortal Wkly Rep* 53(16): 338–343.

Centers for Disease Control and Prevention. (2005). Foodborne Disease Active Surveillance Network (FoodNet) Emerging Infections Program Report on Foodborne Pathogens, 2003. Atlanta: U.S. Department of Health and Human Services.

Cleary, T. G. (2004). The role of Shiga-toxin-producing Escherichia coli in hemorrhagic colitis and hemolytic uremic syndrome. *Semin Pediatr Infect Dis* 15(4): 260–265.

Curriero, F. C., J. A. Patz, et al. (2001). "The association between extreme precipitation and waterborne disease outbreaks in the United States, 1948–1994." *Am J Public Health* 91(8): 1194–1199.

Daniels, N. A., L. MacKinnon, et al. (2000). "Vibrio parahaemolyticus infections in the United States, 1973–1998." *J Infect Dis* 181(5): 1661–1666.

Fisher, IS. (1999) The enter-net international surveillance network—how it works. *Euro Surveill* 4(5): 52–55.

Food Standards Agency. (2002). Measuring foodborne illness levels. United Kingdom: Food Standards Agency.

Gerber, A., H. Karch, et al. (2002). "Clinical course and the role of Shiga toxin-producing *Escherichia coli* infection in the hemolytic-uremic syndrome in pediatric patients, 1997–2000, in Germany and Austria: a prospective study." *J Infect Dis* 186(4): 493–500.

Hardnett, F. P., R. M. Hoekstra, et al. (2004). "Epidemiologic issues in study design and data analysis related to FoodNet activities." *Clin Infect Dis* 38(suppl 3): S121–S126.

Hennessy, T. W., R. Marcus, et al. (2004). "Survey of physician diagnostic practices for patients with acute diarrhea: clinical and public health implications." *Clin Infect Dis* 38(suppl 3): S203–211.

Hlavsa, M. C., J. C. Watson, et al. (2005). "Giardiasis surveillance—United States, 1998–2002." *MMWR Surveill Summ* 54(1): 9–16.

Israelski, D. M., and J. S. Remington (1993). "Toxoplasmosis in patients with cancer." *Clin Infect Dis* 17(suppl 2): S423–S435.

Jones, J. L., A. Lopez, et al. (2004). "Survey of clinical laboratory practices for parasitic diseases." *Clin Infect Dis* 38(suppl 3): S198–S202.

Kendall, P., L. C. Medeiros, et al. (2003). "Food handling behaviors of special importance for pregnant women, infants and young children, the elderly, and immune-compromised people." *J Am Diet Assoc* 103(12): 1646–1649.

Koehler, K. M., T. Lasky, et al. (2006). "Population-based incidence of infection with selected bacterial enteric pathogens in children younger than five years of age, 1996–1998." *Pediatr Infect Dis J* 25(2): 129–134.

Lee, L. A., J. Taylor, G. P. Carter, et al. (1991). "Yersinia enterocolitica O:3 an emerging cause of pediatric gastroenteritis in the United States." The Yersinia enterocolitica collaborative Study Group. *J Infect Dis* 163(3): 660–663

Linnan, M. J., L. Mascola, et al. (1988). "Epidemic listeriosis associated with Mexican-style cheese." *N Engl J Med* 319(13): 823–828.

MacCarthy, N., and J. Giesecke (2001). "Incidence of Guillain-Barre syndrome following infection with *Campylobacter jejuni*." *Am J Epidemiol* 153(6): 610–614.

McAuley, J. B., M. K. Michelson, et al. (1992). "A trichinosis outbreak among Southeast Asian refugees." *Am J Epidemiol* 135(12): 1404–1410.

Mead, P. S., L. Slutsker, et al. (1999). "Food-related illness and death in the United States: reply to Dr. Hedberg." *Emerg Infect Dis* 5(6): 841–842.

Michel, P., J. B. Wilson, et al. (1999). "Temporal and geographical distributions of reported cases of *Escherichia coli* O157:H7 infection in Ontario." *Epidemiol Infect* 122(2): 193–200.

Molina, J., I. Casin, et al. (1995). "Campylobacter infections in HIV-infected patients: clinical and bacteriological features." *AIDS* 9(8): 881–885.

Panackal, A. A., M. M'Ikanatha N, et al. (2002). "Automatic electronic laboratory-based reporting of notifiable infectious diseases at a large health system." *Emerg Infect Dis* 8(7): 685–691.

Ray, S. M., S. D. Ahuja, et al. (2004). "Population-based surveillance for *Yersinia enterocolitica* infections in FoodNet sites, 1996–1999: higher risk of disease in infants and minority populations." *Clin Infect Dis* 38(suppl 3): S181–S189.

Robson, W. L., A. K. Leung, et al. (1991). "Causes of death in hemolytic uremic syndrome." *Child Nephrol Urol* 11(4): 228–233.

Sacktor, N., R. H. Lyles, et al. (2001). "HIV-associated neurologic disease incidence changes: Multicenter AIDS Cohort Study, 1990–1998." *Neurology* 56(2): 257–260.

Schmidt, K., and A. Gervelmeyer. (2003). WHO Surveillance Programme for Control of Foodborne Infections and Intoxications in Europe. Switzerland: United Nations Food and Agriculture Organization/World Health Organization Collaborating Centre for Research and Training in Food Hygiene and Zoonoses.

Selik, R. M., J. M. Karon, et al. (1997). "Effect of the human immunodeficiency virus epidemic on mortality from opportunistic infections in the United States in 1993." *J Infect Dis* 176(3): 632–636.

Selik, R. M., E. T. Starcher, et al. (1987). "Opportunistic diseases reported in AIDS patients: frequencies, associations, and trends." *AIDS* 1(3): 175–182.

Shapiro, R. L., S. Altekruse, et al. (1998). "The role of Gulf Coast oysters harvested in warmer months in *Vibrio vulnificus* infections in the United States, 1988–1996. Vibrio Working Group." *J Infect Dis* 178(3): 752–759.

Smith, J. L. (1999). "Foodborne infections during pregnancy." *J Food Prot* 62(7): 818–829.

Swaminathan, B., T. J. Barrett, S. B. Hunter, R. V. Tauxe, and the CDC PulseNet Task Force (2001). PulseNet: The molecular subtyping network for foodborne bacterial disease surveillance, United States. *Emerg Infect Dis* 7(3): 382–389.

Voetsch, A. C., F. J. Angulo, et al. (2004). "Laboratory practices for stool-specimen culture for bacterial pathogens, including *Escherichia coli* O157:H7, in the FoodNet sites, 1995–2000." *Clin Infect Dis* 38(suppl 3): S190–S197.

4

VEHICLES, SOURCES, RISK FACTORS, AND CAUSES

Tamar Lasky

Epidemiology describes patterns of disease occurrence, with the ultimate purpose of finding an intervention that can prevent the occurrence of illness. We observe the patterns of occurrence and then take action: modify the water supply, boil the milk, improve the diet, remove lead from gasoline. Before we take action, we subject our observations to criteria to evaluate whether we have identified an intervention that will yield our desired goal of preventing the disease in question. These criteria help us decide whether or not observed relationships between two events are causal.

Epidemiologic thinking about causality has undergone changes over the past century; however, ideas about causality have often been presented as static absolutes. Furthermore, ideas about causality have been shaped by the types of diseases of concern in a given decade. This is especially relevant to epidemiologists working on food safety in the twenty-first century, because the epidemiology of food-borne illness draws on infectious disease methods developed in the 1950s (and earlier) and chronic disease methods developed in the 1950s, 1960s, and 1970s. The two epidemiologies coexist in an uneasy mixture of terminology and assumptions about causality.

Many readers of this book will have read extensively about causality and related philosophical thinking, and it is not my purpose here to recapitulate the broad range of thinking on causality. The purpose of this discussion is to highlight aspects of epidemiologic causal thinking that are relevant to the way that food safety issues are addressed in the present. The key points are that present thinking incorporates concepts from two different eras in epidemiology, that the inconsistencies between these two views have not been entirely worked out, and that we are not always aware of the concepts or assumptions at play in the food safety arena.

The Infectious Disease Causal Model

During the late nineteenth century, germ theory and the emergence of microbiology established that microscopic living organisms caused diseases and that different organisms were associated with different diseases. From the late nineteenth century through the first few decades of the twentieth century, epidemiology was most notably preoccupied with identifying the individual organisms causing different diseases in humans, animals, and even plants, and a progression of discoveries announced the causes of anthrax, pear blight, gonorrhea, malaria, tuberculosis, diphtheria, gangrene, babesiosis, bubonic plague—each cause being a unique living organism. These were followed by discoveries identifying vectors carrying the living organisms—ticks, flies, rodents, and so on. Infectious disease epidemiology concentrated on the isolation of pathogens and identification of vectors and routes of transmission.

Robert Koch (who first isolated the organism causing anthrax, and then the organism causing tuberculosis) recognized that finding the organism in the presence of disease was not sufficient for demonstrating causality:

> The most skeptical can raise the objection that the discovered microorganism is not the cause but only an accompaniment of the disease. However, many times this objection has a certain validity, and then it is necessary to obtain a perfect proof to satisfy oneself that the parasite (his word) and the disease are not only correlated, but actually causally related, and that the parasite is the actual cause of the disease. (Koch 1884)

He developed his thinking further and built on earlier work by Jakob Henle, yielding four postulates guiding the microbiological concept of causality:

1. The microorganism must be present in every case of the disease.
2. The microorganism must be isolated from the diseased host and grown in pure culture.
3. The specific disease must be reproduced when a pure culture of the microorganism is inoculated into a healthy susceptible host.

4. The microorganism must be recoverable from the experimentally infected host.

These postulates were eventually applied to all infectious diseases, bacterial, parasitic, and viral, even though Koch was not aware of the distinctions between bacteria, parasites, and viruses when he developed the postulates. The postulates provided a starting point, but even within the world of infectious diseases, the recognition grew that the postulates cannot always be applied rigidly. A bacterium that is part of the normal flora may become a pathogen in certain situations: if it acquires extra virulence factors making it pathogenic; if it gains access to deep tissues by trauma, surgery, or insertion of intravascular lines; or if the patients are immunocompromised. Further, not all of those infected or colonized by a pathogenic bacterium will develop disease—subclinical infection may occur, and despite Koch's postulates, some bacteria are not culturable *in vitro* or there may be no suitable animal model of infection. Nonetheless, Koch's postulates form the basis for any discussion of infectious disease causality, microbiology, and infectious disease epidemiology.

Infectious Disease Epidemiologic Concepts

In addition to the Koch-Henle postulates and the concept of causality, infectious disease epidemiology contributed related concepts, such as vehicle, vector, source, reservoirs, and zoonosis. Some of these concepts are closely related to each other: a vector is a living carrier (insect, rodent, bird, etc.) that transports an infectious agent from an infected individual to a susceptible individual. The vehicle of transmission can be a vector, or it can be food, person to person, or some other mode. A reservoir of infection can be animal, insect or human; the organism serving as a reservoir may or may not also be the vector. Some diseases, zoonoses, are shared by humans and animals. Sometimes, human susceptibility to a disease is not revealed until humans and animals interact: weather, population growth, migration, and other factors can bring humans and animals into closer contact with each other, resulting in infections of humans with previously unheard of illnesses. Hanta virus and monkey pox are recent examples of this phenomenon. These concepts are important because factors affecting reservoirs, vehicles, vectors, and so forth, can affect incidence of disease but may not be "causes" in traditional infectious disease causal thinking. The pathogen itself is the cause, but factors affecting exposure to the pathogen contribute to the occurrence of disease. As discussed below, multicausal concepts of disease developed in the epidemiology of chronic disease permit us to consider factors that affect reservoirs, vehicles, vectors, and the occurrence of disease.

The Chronic Disease Concept of Risk Factors

When physicians and epidemiologists turned their attention to chronic diseases such as heart disease and cancer, they naturally brought with them the concepts of causality learned in studying infectious diseases, but very quickly found them ill-adapted to their needs. By the 1940s and 1950s, it was clear that smoking appeared to cause lung cancer, but also appeared to cause heart disease. This defied Koch's postulate that the causal agent results in the same disease after it is introduced to a new host. Some people developed heart disease or cancer without ever having smoked. Again, this defied Koch's postulate that the causal agent be present in all cases of the disease. Koch's postulates did not fit because multiple factors contribute to the development of heart disease and cancer. A factor may be one of several contributing to the ultimate development of the disease, and it might not even be necessary for the development of disease. Other combinations of factors could also lead to the same disease.

Leading epidemiologists in the 1950s began discussing new concepts of causality, and ultimately, Austin Bradford Hill published criteria for causality in 1965 (Hill 1965). These criteria had already been incorporated into the 1964 report released by the U.S. Surgeon General, which concluded, "Smoking is causally related to lung cancer" (U.S. Department of Health, Education, and Welfare 1964). This is a long way from the announcement that the tubercle bacillus, *Mycobacterium tuberculosis*, causes tuberculosis. The language changed subtly from "A causes B" to "A is causally related to B." The Bradford Hill criteria included the strength of association, consistency of study findings, specificity of the relationship between exposure and disease, relationship in time, biological gradient, biological plausibility, coherence of the evidence, experimental evidence, and analogy. More important, the assessment of causality involved a weighing of a body of information from different sources and, unlike Koch's postulates, did not require all criteria to be met. Hill himself pointed out that circumstances would arise when all criteria could not be met.

The wording used by the Surgeon General, "causally related," seems to invite more possibilities than the more direct usage, "causes." It implies that a factor can contribute to development of a condition but may not be necessary or sufficient for every occurrence of the condition. From this multicausal concept of disease, it was a small step to the concept of risk factors. As defined by Last (1995), a risk factor may have any of the following meanings:

- An attribute or exposure that is associated with an increased probability of a specified outcome . . . not necessarily a causal factor
- An attribute or exposure that increases the probability of occurrence of disease or other specified outcome

- A determinant that can be modified by intervention, thereby reducing the probability of occurrence of disease or other specified outcomes

These definitions seem to be semantic hair-splitting: risk factors—not necessarily a causal factor? Then what do they do, how do they act? I prefer to focus on those that are contributory factors, suggesting that they play a mechanistic role in modifying the risk of disease, whereas the term "risk factor" in the definitions above includes markers of risk, and covariates of causal variables, a broader group of variables. Nonetheless, the term "risk factor" is an integral part of epidemiology and, interestingly enough, has become an integral part of the epidemiology of food-borne illnesses.

Causality in an Outbreak Setting

When an outbreak is recognized, public health officials generally identify the pathogen early in the investigation: in recent years, pulsed-field gel electrophoresis typing may identify a pathogen causing an outbreak before an outbreak is even recognized in any other way. Identification of the causal agent does not complete the work of the outbreak epidemiologist, although it is a necessary and important first step. It is also important to find out what foods were contaminated, how the pathogen was introduced to the food, and what errors in food handling occurred, to ensure that further illnesses will not occur.

In the traditional infectious disease concept of causality, the pathogen is the "cause" of the illnesses and outbreak, but we are still interested in knowing the factors that caused the contamination or exposure. These factors can be termed "risk factors," "contributing factors," "factors causing exposure," or simply "causes," and we can borrow from chronic disease epidemiology to think of food-borne outbreak as a multicausal event resulting from a series of events leading to introduction of pathogens into a food product and human exposure to disease-causing pathogens.

The "farm-to-table" continuum describes the series of opportunities for contamination and pathogen multiplication from growing animals and plants for food to processing agricultural products, manufacturing and transporting foods, preparing foods for consumption, and eating foods (figure 4-1). Each outbreak is a result of an error or series of errors along the continuum where pathogens are introduced, efforts to eliminate pathogens fail, or improper handling allows pathogens to multiply (tables 4-1, 4-2). After an outbreak, one identifies the errors leading to that particular outbreak and takes steps to see that the same error does not occur again. Thus, the epidemiologist will need to identify the pathogen, the food vehicle, and the factors contributing to the occurrence of the pathogen on the food vehicle.

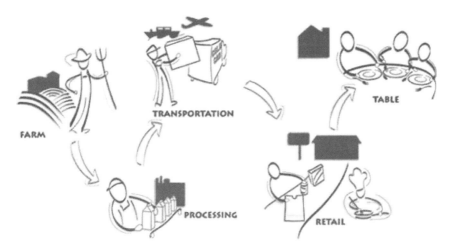

Figure 4-1. The farm-to-table continuum. Opportunities to prevent or cause illness occur at any point along the continuum. Source: Center for Food Safety and Nutrition, FDA.

Causality in Assessing Risk Factors Contributing to Overall Levels of Illness

The farm-to-table continuum that is assessed in an individual outbreak is also assessed when policy makers and public health officials look to intervene and lower the overall levels of food-borne illnesses. Each individual outbreak provides anecdotal evidence of steps that can go wrong, and after reviewing a number of outbreak investigations, one sees that errors may occur anywhere and everywhere along the farm-to-table continuum. We would like to be able to evaluate the relative contribution of each factor along the continuum and identify points for effective intervention. Although many measures are in place along the continuum, it is important to know where to strengthen measures and where to remove ineffective measures. Most food safety measures involve some cost in terms of equipment, labor, price to the consumer, taste, and appeal; thus, there is an upper limit on the number of food safety measures that can be added to a system. It is necessary to be able to measure the effect of an intervention on food safety and quantify that effect in terms of illness and mortality averted in order to justify any costs associated with implementation. From this perspective, interventions or food safety measures can be considered "risk factors" as defined by Last (1995): "A determinant that can be modified by intervention, thereby reducing the probability of occurrence of disease or other specified outcomes" (p. 148). Disentangling the many contributory factors and identifying key points for intervention will be major challenges for epidemiologists interested in promoting food safety measures aimed at decreasing the incidence of food-borne illness.

TABLE 4-1   The farm-to-table continuum and control of food-borne pathogens

Contamination Source	Introduction of Pathogens	Failure to Eliminate Pathogens	Allowing Pathogens to Multiply
Farm			
Health of workers Water supply for plants and animals Handling of animal waste Health of animals	Sick workers can contaminate fruit and vegetables. Contaminated water can contaminate fruit and vegetables. Farming practices can affect prevalence of infected animals or the typical bacterial flora.	Animal handling practices can fail to isolate, treat, or remove infected animals.	Climate, stagnant water supplies
Processing			
Health of workers Crowding Slaughter practices HACCP* practices	Sick workers can contaminate plant and animal products and machinery. Improper processing can lead to cross-contamination and introduction of fecal matter to foods.	Inadequate rinsing or omission of other steps can leave pathogens on products. Inadequate heating processes can fail to eliminate pathogens.	Inadequate cooling processes can allow pathogens to multiply.
Transportation	Improperly cleaned trucks can introduce pathogens from previous shipments to subsequent shipments (e.g., Salmonella and ice cream).		Refrigeration in trucks or train cars can fail and allow pathogens to multiply.
Preparation and food handling			
Health of food workers Cleanliness of plant, kitchen Heating, refrigeration capabilities	Sick workers can introduce viral, bacterial, and other pathogens to foods. Improperly maintained vent and air conditioning systems can contaminate food products. Improper handling can cross-contaminate food that will not be cooked.	Inadequate heating and/or cooking can fail to kill pathogens.	Inadequate heating or refrigeration can allow pathogens to multiply.

*Hazard Analysis and Critical Control Points.

TABLE 4-2   The farm-to-table continuum and control of antibiotic resistance, chemicals and metals, and genetically modified foods

Contamination Source	Antibiotic Use	Chemicals, Pesticides, and Heavy Metals	Genetically Modified Foods
Farm	Use of antibiotics in animal feed	Additives to feed Pesticide use	Mixing seeds from different batches
Processing		Preservatives Additives Industrial chemicals	Mixing products from different farms, processing lines, or lots
Preparation		Preservatives Additives Industrial, cleaning chemicals, other	Mixing products

While we know the specific factors leading to specific food-borne outbreaks, it is more difficult to quantify the contribution of factors to overall levels of food-borne illness. As described in the following chapters, efforts to improve food safety are directed at all points along the farm-to-table continuum. Veterinarians and agriculture experts focus on ways to improve the health of animals and improve hygiene in slaughter and processing. Regulatory agencies target steps along the continuum, and economists model and project the costs of changes in the manufacturing, processing, distribution, labeling, and marketing of foods. Environmental sanitarians work to identify factors that lead to a work environment favorable to safe food preparation in retail settings, nursing homes, and private homes.

The role of epidemiologists at the aggregate level is to integrate the various perspectives and to apply epidemiologic principles to measure and assess the various factors affecting introduction and multiplication of pathogens, and failure to eliminate pathogens, from farm to table. This is not a simple extension of the role of an epidemiologist in an outbreak investigation, but more closely resembles the role of chronic disease epidemiologists who carefully disentangle the many factors affecting, for example, cardiovascular mortality —population factors, lifestyle factors, hospital practices, medication practices, and so forth. At the aggregate level, food-borne illnesses can be thought of as a multicausal disease (or group of diseases), with common threads leading to a common result, food-borne illness, but many diverse causal pathways, as well. For the epidemiologist engaged in such work, it is important to understand the differences in approaches required for the acute, outbreak situation compared to the overall, aggregate situation. For the nonepidemiologist working with epidemiologists, it is important to be aware that two lines of epidemiologic thinking have developed over almost a century, one from infectious disease epidemiology, and one from chronic disease epidemiology, and that both are essential to the prevention and control of food-borne illness today.

Beyond Infectious Disease

As stated in chapter 1, concerns about food safety span a number of issues beyond illness from infection with a food-borne pathogen. Very closely related to the issue of infection is the acquisition of antibiotic-resistant strains of bacteria. A food-borne outbreak of antibiotic-resistant bacteria further complicates treatment and raises the level of concern about infection. This situation falls under the same causal principles governing any food-borne outbreak of an infectious disease. However, on the aggregate level, the replacement of one population of bacteria by another population, with increasing proportions of resistant bacteria as well as resistance to an increased number of antibiotics, is a food safety issue that takes on an ecologic breadth not readily addressed by the principles discussed above. Genetic and evolutionary principles need to be applied in attempting to identify the causes, risk factors, and/or contributory factors leading to changes in the prevalence of antibiotic-resistant bacteria in our food and water supply, and ultimately in human illness. The food safety community has not yet fully engaged this issue, but data collected to monitor food-borne infections are beginning to be used to describe and document the progressive change in our microbial populations. Some tools from the epidemiology of food-borne illness can be applied to the problem of antibiotic-resistant bacteria, but much more is needed in this arena.

Food can become contaminated by materials other than living pathogens— pesticides, industrial oils and solvents, metals, and other contaminants can enter the food supply at any point along the farm-to-table continuum, entering animal feed, grinding, and processing mixtures and prepared food. A major difference from the issue of living organisms lies in the fact that many potential contaminants are used deliberately as part of agriculture, food production, and food processing. Accidental contamination, such as the spilling of a chemical into feed or leakage of machine oil into a meat grinding vat, can result in illness and complaints resembling an infectious food-borne disease outbreak (people begin calling and reporting complaints, symptoms, and illnesses to stores and health authorities), and many chemicals and pesticides are used in agriculture at low levels and over wide ranges of products. The acute outbreak model from infectious food-borne illness applies readily to the causal model of an outbreak resulting from acute contamination with chemicals or metals. The contaminant enters at various points along the farm-to-table continuum and results in illness among those exposed to the foods containing the contaminant. For example, aldicarb, a cholinesterase-inhibiting pesticide, has been associated with several outbreaks (Centers for Disease Control and Prevention 1986, 1999). In the most recent report, it appeared that the pesticide had been placed in a can labeled "black pepper" by a crawfish farmer (Centers for Disease Control and Prevention 1999). A relative found the can and used it when preparing cabbage salad for a company lunch. As a result, 10 of 20 people attending the lunch sought emergency care. In 1985, watermelons and cantaloupes in California were apparently contaminated on the farm with aldicarb, resulting in widespread reports of illness (Centers for Disease Control and Prevention 1986). A total of 692 probable cases were reported in California. Although investigators identified fields thought to be contaminated, melons from different farms were so intermingled in the distribution chain that all watermelons in the distribution chain had to be destroyed.

Low levels of pesticides and chemical residues are permitted in agricultural products and foods based on analysis and regulation by a number of federal agencies, including the U.S. Environmental Protection Agency, Food and Drug Administration (FDA), and U.S. Department of Agriculture (USDA). These are also regulated to some degree at an international level to promote trade of agricultural products. The safety levels agreed upon are based on varying levels of data and on risk assessments, where possible, but as with any process, they are subject to questioning and revision. New data, changes in eating habits, and changes in consumer preferences all could generate debate on the acceptability of safety levels and guidelines; epidemiologic data would be a key part of such a debate and would draw heavily on principles developed in environmental epidemiology. At the same time, causal pathways identified in studying food-borne infections might also be relevant to understanding the pathways by which individual pesticide and chemical residues reach the consumer.

A fascinating causal pathway proceeds from the ingredients in animal feed to the presence of contaminants in food products from the animal. The transmission of *Trichinella* cysts from garbage, feces, and rodents eaten by pigs was identified as a cause of trichinosis in humans and resulted in regulations (early in the 20th century) requiring that garbage be boiled before it is fed to pigs raised for human consumption. More recently, we recognized that feed containing ground-up beef proteins, particularly from the nervous system, was capable of transmitting prions when fed to cattle, and the prions could in turn infect humans who consumed the beef products. This particular pathway, from animal feed to animal to human consuming the animal, also results in the transmission of noninfective agents. For example, antibiotics containing arsenic are fed to chickens to prevent infections; arsenic can then be found in the chicken eaten by humans, resulting in arsenic exposure to humans consuming the chickens.

When pesticides and chemicals are used in the growing and manufacturing of food, the epidemiologist does not necessarily need to identify the chemical or the point of entry, as in an outbreak situation. Instead, the epidemiologic role may be that of exposure assessment: measurement of the amounts of chemicals in the food ingested by consumers. As mentioned, many pharmaceuticals are used in raising animals, and among them are arsenic-containing additives meant to control intestinal parasites in chickens. The FDA requires specific periods of time for drugs to be withheld before slaughter of the animal, and the USDA Food Safety and Inspection Service collects samples of animals to measure residues remaining in the slaughtered animals. The program is an enforcement tool to make sure that farmers follow the withdrawal period required by the FDA. The samples of data are analyzed chemically for content, but the resultant databases are analyzed categorically (violations and nonviolations).

An epidemiologist approaching the data will first quantify levels of chemical or residue detected and then use the data to estimate doses delivered to consumers of the animal product. This was done by Lasky et al. (2004) to estimate arsenic concentrations in chicken. The quantitative analysis of arsenic concentrations permits the epidemiologist to assess the potential hazard of a particular practice at a specific point along the farm-to-table continuum. In this instance, the practice of feeding arsenic-containing additives to poultry can be assessed relative to its benefits (fewer infected chickens) and hazards (increasing concentrations of arsenic in chicken). Although the hazardous nature of arsenic has been established, study of the practice of feeding arsenic-containing additives is still required. The amount and distribution of arsenic in chicken products and the patterns of consumption (how many people eat how much chicken?) are classic exposure measurement questions. This information needs to be considered in light of information about effects of cooking and metabolism and absorption of arsenic, and epidemiologic studies might be needed to correlate exposure to arsenic through chicken consumption and health effects, such as cancer. Because there is a large body of information about arsenic and cancer, risk assessors might be able to estimate the expected health effects of arsenic consumption through chicken. Thus, for practices that deliberately introduce chemicals or pesticides at any point along the farm-to-table continuum, epidemiologic methods can be used to estimate exposure while drawing on causal evidence from other fields, most notable, environmental and occupational epidemiology. This information, in turn, can be used by risk assessors to estimate potential risk.

Another type of contamination could be the mixture of genetically modified foods with non-genetically modified foods. Consumers currently expect genetically modified food products to be labeled and separated from non-genetically modified food products to permit individual discretion in the purchase of either group of products. When genetically modified foods become mixed with non-genetically modified food products, they are considered to be contaminants of the food. The contamination is analogous to that with pathogens or with chemicals: contamination can take place anywhere along the farm-to-table continuum.

The farm-to-table continuum serves as a framework for considering points of intervention and opportunities to improve food safety. In an acute outbreak, we are concerned with identification of the specific hazard causing the outbreak and the point at which a hazard was introduced or was not contained. From a more general perspective, we are concerned with weighing the relative contribution of factors along the farm-to-table continuum to the occurrence of food-borne illness. This expands our concept of causal factors well beyond the pathogen or chemical contaminant to include farming practices, slaughter and production, and food handling in restaurants and in the home. The contaminant itself, whether infectious or not, is the immediate cause of illness; factors leading to contamination are also "causes" of food-borne illness, because prevention and control of food-borne illness depend on identification of factors leading to contamination and elimination of contaminants that may be there. These issues are addressed further in chapters 9–13 on risk assessment, economic analysis, food production, and regulatory issues.

References

Centers for Disease Control and Prevention. (1986). "Epidemiologic Notes and Reports Aldicarb Food Poisoning from Contaminated Melons—California." *Morbidity and Mortality Weekly Reports* 35(16): 254–258.

Centers for Disease Control and Prevention. (1999). "Aldicarb as a Cause of Food Poisoning—Louisiana, 1998." *Morbidity and Mortality Weekly Reports* 48(13): 269–271.

Hill, A. B. (1965). "The Environment and Disease: Association or Causation?" *Proceedings of the Royal Society of Medicine* 58: 295–300.

Koch, R. (1884). Die Aetiologie der Tuberkulose. In: *Milestones in Microbiology: 1556 to 1940.* (1998) T. D. Brock, editor. Washington, DC, American Society for Microbiology Press: 116–118. (Originally published 1884.)

Lasky, T., W. Sun, et al. (2004). "Mean Total Arsenic Concentrations in Chicken 1989–2000 and Estimated Exposures for Consumers of Chicken." *Environ Health Perspect* 112(1): 18–21.

Last, J. M. (1995). *A Dictionary of Epidemiology*. New York, Oxford University Press.

U.S. Department of Health, Education, and Welfare. (1964). Smoking and Health: Report of the Advisory Committee to the Surgeon General of the Public Health Service. Public Health Service Publication No. 1103. Washington, DC, U.S. Government Printing Office.

5

FOOD AS EXPOSURE: MEASURING DIETARY INTAKES AND CONSUMPTION PATTERNS

Nga L. Tran and Leila Barraj

Dietary exposure assessment is the process of evaluating human exposure to a chemical, microbiological, or physical agent present in foods. Dietary exposure assessment draws on a highly developed methodology that nutritionists, dieticians, and biochemists have used for more than 60 years. With respect to food safety, dietary exposure assessment is a tool for estimating intake for the purposes of risk assessment. It also identifies foods causally associated with an acute outbreak; however, the more sophisticated methodologies of dietary exposure assessment are rarely part of an outbreak investigation. Although this chapter focuses on uses in risk assessment, there is a great need to draw on these methodologies in outbreak investigations. More discussion of this issue appears toward the end of the chapter. Within the field of dietary risk assessment, direct and indirect approaches are possible. Direct methods estimate the intake of individuals within a population subgroup. Indirect methods combine food consumption data with contaminant concentration data derived from two different data sources.

Methods for direct assessment include a chemical analysis of duplicate samples of all foods and beverages consumed. For example, in a duplicate diet study, participants prepare, record, weigh (optional), and retain portions of each food and beverage they consume during each day of the study period. Duplicate portions are generally collected for one day, but multiple days will

76

offer a better description of the individual's contaminant intake, since dietary intake varies from day to day. In some cases, duplicate diet samples are collected from the same individuals at different times of the year to assess seasonal intake variability.

The duplicate portion method was used in the assessment of human exposure to benzo(a)pyrene via food ingestion in the Total Human Environmental Exposure Study (Waldman et al., 1991). Twenty individuals participated in the study and collected duplicate portions of the foods they consumed over three periods of 14 days each. Fujita and Morikawa (1992) used the method to assess regional differences in dietary intakes of environmental pollutants in Japan. One hundred twenty-seven women in five cities participated in the study and collected duplicate samples of all foods consumed in a typical day.

In the indirect method, the likelihood or prevalence of an agent (chemical, microbiological, or physical) and the concentration(s) of that agent in food(s) are first estimated and then combined with food consumption to estimate intakes of the agent of interest. Dietary intake of a food component, such as a micronutrient; a food ingredient, such as a food additive; or a contaminant, such as a pesticide residue, is often indirectly estimated based on two parameters: (1) the concentration of the food component, ingredient, or contaminant at the time of consumption (C_f = mg/kg food) and (2) the amount of the food consumed (L = kg food/day). To account for dietary intake of a food component, ingredient, or contaminant from the consumption of multiple foods, the following equation applies:

$$E_t = \sum_i (C_f)_i (L)_i \tag{1}$$

where i is the number of different food types consumed, C_f is the concentration of the component, ingredient, or contaminant in the foods (mg/kg), and L is the amount of food consumed (kg/day). Under this general framework, exposure to a food component can be estimated as either the product of an average consumption of a food and an average concentration of the food component, ingredient, or contaminant in or on that food or the product of the probability distributions of food intakes and component, ingredient, or contaminant concentrations.

Food Intake Assessment

Food production statistics, food consumption surveys, retail food purchase data, and household surveys may be useful in providing data regarding food production or food consumption. Food production statistics provide an estimate of the amount of food available to the total population. They are generally compiled and reported for raw or semiprocessed agricultural commodities, and they represent the total annual amount of a commodity available for domestic consumption. Food consumption is expressed as the total annual quantity of food available for each person in the total population (per capita amount). The daily per-capita amount may be calculated by dividing the annual amount by 365. Examples of this type of data include the United Nations Food and Agriculture Organization's Food Balance Sheets and other national statistics on food production, disappearance, or utilization. Because these data are available for most countries and are compiled and reported consistently across countries, they can be useful in conducting exposure assessments at the international level.

Retail food purchase data provide detailed information about specific food products, which is often lacking from food consumption surveys. They are typically at the household level and thus do not describe the amount of food actually consumed by specific individuals or who is consuming them. However, the information can be combined with other food consumption data to refine the characterization of food consumption.

Household surveys may include questions such as what foods are available in the household; what foods enter the household; whether the foods were purchased, grown, or obtained some other way; and what foods are used up by the household. Surveys may ask respondents to maintain food records, recall food eaten in a 24-hour period, provide estimates on food frequency questionnaires, or provide dietary histories (Pao and Cypel, 1990, as cited in Life Science Research Office, 1993). Individual food intake surveys are estimates of food consumption by specific individuals.

Food consumption surveys can be conducted at the national level or for specific subpopulations, such as people residing in particular regions, of specific age groups, or with specific occupations. Surveys designed to determine food consumption patterns over a longer time frame (weeks to months for each survey participant) usually determine not the specific quantity of food consumed but rather only the frequency of consumption.

Food intakes may be current or from the immediate, recent, or distant past. Survey methods to collect food consumption data can be retrospective, for example, the 24-hour or other short-term recalls, food frequencies, and diet histories; or prospective, for example, food diaries and food records or duplicate portions. Survey methods such as food records, 24-hour recalls, and food frequency questionnaires are described below.

Food Records   The subject or a designated surrogate keeps a food record for a specified time period. This method relies on either weighed or estimated records. With weighed records, subjects are taught to weigh and record foods immediately before eating and to weigh any leftover. Scales and record books are used. With estimated records, subjects are taught to keep records of portion sizes that are described as household measures, for example, spoons or ladles. Estimated records are less cumbersome than weighed records; however, a loss of accuracy is more likely to occur with estimated records (Willett, 1990; Cameron, 1988). In general, the food record method is effective when the surveyed population is literate, motivated, and cooperative. Since the burden on the participants is large, subject cooperation and record validity may decline in relation to the length of the recording process. In addition, the process of writing the record can cause a change in food intake through self-observation and awareness, by omission of eating to avoid the bothersome detail of measuring and writing, or by avoiding a normally consumed food because of embarrassment about reporting it. Furthermore, delay in recording meals and snacks can affect accuracy in quantification as well as memory of foods consumed (Willett, 1990).

24-Hour Recall Survey   This method is most commonly used to collect food intake information (Life Science Research Office, 1993). Under this approach, a trained interviewer asks the respondent to recall information about the foods and the amounts of foods he or she has eaten in a 24-hour period. The respondent is asked to describe the food eaten in detail, including the type and amount of food, brand name, method of preparation, and so forth. This method can be administered in person or over the telephone for the duration of approximately 20–30 minutes. The main advantage with this method is that it does not pose a large burden on participants and does not require that the survey participants be literate (Willett, 1990).

Food Frequency Questionnaires   Qualitative food frequency methods are often used in epidemiology studies to obtain information on usual food intake over an extended period of time to assess diet and disease relationships (Pao and Cypel, 1990, as cited in Life Science Research Office, 1993). This method focuses on average long-term diet, such as intake over weeks, months, or years. Respondents are asked to report the number of times each food on a checklist is eaten during a specified period. These checklists vary in the number of foods included and the specificity of the description, for example, fruits in general versus apples and oranges in particular. Food frequency questionnaires are practical in epidemiological applications because they are self-administered (Willett, 1990). However, because this method is qualitative and foods are broadly aggregated into groups, data from food frequency questionnaires have had limited use in quantitative exposure assessments.

U.S. National Food Consumption Surveys

The U.S. Department of Agriculture (USDA) and the National Center of Health Statistics (NCHS) have conducted nationwide food consumption surveys, including the USDA Continuing Survey of Food Intakes by Individuals

(CSFII) for 1985–1986, 1989–1990, 1990–1991, 1994–1996, and 1998; the Nationwide Food Consumption Survey (NFCS) for 1987–1988; and the NCHS National Health and Nutrition Examination Survey (NHANES) for 1999+. Risk assessors have relied extensively on consumption data from these nationwide consumption surveys for risk assessment.

USDA Surveys

The USDA's survey sample was drawn from all private households and designed to provide a multistage stratified area probability sample representative of the 48 contiguous states. The stratification plan took into account geographic location, degree of urbanization, and socioeconomic status. The 48 states were grouped into nine census geographic divisions, and then all land areas within the divisions were divided into three urbanization classifications: central city, suburban, and nonmetropolitan. Each successive sampling stage selected increasingly smaller, more specific locations.

The 1987–1988 NFCS is a national food consumption survey that collected food consumption data during home visits by trained interviewers using an interviewer-administered 24-hour dietary recall for the day preceding the interview, and a self-administered two-day dietary record for the day of the interview and the following day. Thus, three consecutive days of intake were recorded.

The 1989–1991 CSFII is part of the USDA's three-year CSFII cycle. Similar to the 1987–1988 NFCS, food consumption data were also collected during home visits by trained interviewers using an interviewer-administered 24-hour dietary recall for the day preceding the interview, and a self-administered two-day dietary record for the day of the interview and the following day. The number of person days included in this survey is 31,149.

The diet of adult women 19–50 years of age and their preschoolers 1–5 years of age was the focus of the 1985–1986 CSFII. An initial group of 1,459 women and their 489 children were asked to provide dietary data for six nonconsecutive days at approximately two-month intervals over a one-year period between April 1985 and March 1986. Data for the first day were collected by personal interview and on the following days by telephone. Not all participants completed all six days. Three or more days were completed by 333 children and 1,127 women (National Resource Defense Council, 1989). Consumption data from the 1994–1996 CSFII and the 1998 Supplemental Children's Survey (U.S. Department of Agriculture, 1999) are for the most recent two nonconsecutive days of food intake.

National Health and Nutrition Examination Survey (NHANES)

The purpose of NHANES is to assess the health and nutritional status of children and adults living in the United States.

The nutrition assessment tools used in NHANES were designed to provide monitoring data enabling the assessment of the nutritional status of the population over time, reference data for nutritional biochemistries, anthropometric data and nutrient intakes, and data for research to examine relationships between diet and health. NHANES 1999+ is an annual, cross-sectional survey that is based on a complex multistage cluster survey design to collect information about the health and diet of the civilian, noninstitutionalized populations of the United States. NHANES also annually collects information about the frequency of consumption for a subset of foods. NHANES samples about 5,000 people every year through a Mobile Examination Center, which travels around the country to randomly selected households, conducting both interviews and physical exams. The surveys conduct both in-home interviews and physical examinations focusing on several population groups and health topics. Some of the population groups include the general U.S. population, adults 18–79 years of age, infants, children 6–11 years of age, youths 12–17 years of age, adolescents 15–19 years of age, pregnant women, African Americans, and Hispanic Americans. Some of the health topics include risk factors (e.g., smoking, alcohol consumption, sexual practices, drug use, physical fitness), reproductive health, cardio-vascular disease, mental health, nutrition, oral health, and vision.

Consumption Data Selection

Consumption data, such as those derived from USDA's 1989–1992 CSFII, the Australian National Survey (Australia New Zealand Food Authority, 1997), the U.K. national surveys for adults and for toddlers, and other European surveys (Scientific Committee on Foods Intake and Exposure Working Group, 1994; DAFNE II, 1995) are available for many countries. The available data may be quite different, depending upon how and when they were collected (Petersen and Douglass, 1994; Trichopoulou and Lagiou, 1997). There are a number of specific survey design questions to consider when selecting food consumption data to estimate exposure (see table 5-1).

The best data set for each intake analysis will depend upon the question to be answered and the population for whom the estimates are to be made. When using data from consumption surveys, it is necessary to infer information from a sample of the population and to apply that to the total population. To do so, it must be confirmed that the sample is representative of the population; if not, statistical weights could be used to make the results representative. Specifically, assumptions must be made regarding how well the survey period represents a person's eating pattern. It may also be appropriate to incorporate measures that will account for day-to-day variability.

When food frequency data are used, it may be necessary to make special adjustments to reflect the differences in the level of detail in the surveys. Food

TABLE 5-1   Food consumption survey design questions

Was the survey designed to permit high data flexibility with little weighting?
Does it contain relatively few nonrespondents or other statistical problems?
Was design and survey methodology validated?
When (how long ago) were the data collected?
Are current patterns of consumption of the foods of interest similar?
For which country or countries do the data apply?
Does it incorporate food source, brand names, and packaging information?
Are there adequate numbers of respondents?
Are food descriptions completed (form [e.g., raw, processed], level of detail, brand names)?
For which population were the food consumption data collected (age, sex, ethnicity)?
For which geographical regions?
Were data collected during all seasons?
What foods were included?
Was the quantity of each food estimated?

groups that are most appropriate for evaluating novel foods may be different from those traditionally used to estimate nutrient intake. For example, it may be necessary to match the survey food groups to data on composition for individual foods within these groups. Some foods may be consumed both as discrete items and as components of combination foods or food mixtures. Therefore, most evaluations will need to incorporate estimates for ingredients derived from commodities that are subsequently found in a large variety of food products. For example, corn may be consumed as a single food item or can be consumed as a component of a casserole. As another example, milk may be consumed as a beverage or as an ingredient (often in very small amounts) in many food items.

Food consumption surveys of individuals are frequently conducted for the purpose of assessing the nutritional status of a population rather than to characterize consumption of specific foods. Although these surveys may provide information about consumption by specific age/gender groups, they may not describe foods in sufficient detail or include enough participants from sensitive subpopulations or even collect information necessary to identify these subpopulations. Raw data from the surveys are not always available, and the risk assessor must rely on aggregated data, which may limit the usefulness of the data.

In summary, traditional food consumption surveys are useful to predict dietary intake of foods, food ingredients, and nutrients. The same databases can also be used to assure that no nutritional deficiency is introduced as a result of the proposed modification by comparing intakes of nutrients under a variety of different scenarios or by comparing nutritional intakes from the new foods to those from the foods that are being replaced.

Estimating Food Intakes

There are many ways by which both consumption amount and frequency of consumption may be calculated, each resulting in different values and representing a different characterization of food consumption. In the case of chemical contaminants, the toxicological profile of the contaminants guides the choice of the method used to estimate intake. For instance, for contaminants with acute effects, daily intake estimates or intakes per meal are more relevant than intakes over a period of time (Rees and Tennant, 1993). Also, there may be instances when intake from a single food is desired (e.g., because it is the only food likely to contain the contaminant), and others where intake from several foods or the entire diet is of interest.

Per-Capita and Per-User Consumption

Quantitative daily food consumption surveys such as 24-hour recall result in a database of people reporting consuming a food (users) and people who did not report a food intake (nonusers). If the 24-hour recall day is truly a representative day, the nonusers can be assumed to have zero consumption. However, it is impossible to ascertain if it is a representative day and if nonusers are true noneaters (i.e., never eat or true zero intake). Two measures of intakes can be derived. The per-capita estimate is calculated by dividing the total amount of food available to (or consumed by) the population by the total number of people in the population. This reflects the amount of the food available to the total population although not necessarily the amount of the food actually consumed by an individual. Per-user consumption is calculated by dividing the total amount of food by the number of people who reported eating the food. These measures need to be defined by a unit of time—is the consumption estimate per year, per day, or per eating occasion?

Point Estimate or Distribution Estimate?

Another issue to consider is whether a point estimate or distribution should be used. People obviously do not all eat the same amount of each food, nor do they eat the same amount of food every day. It will be necessary to determine whether the most appropriate metric is a point estimate, or whether to characterize the intra- and interindividual variability. And, if a point estimate is to be used, should it represent the "average" consumer, or should it represent the high-end consumer?

Frequency of Consumption

The frequency of consumption may refer to the proportion of the population that consumes a food and/or how often an individual consumes a food over a specific period of time. This information can be derived from food consumption surveys and other sources such as food frequency questionnaires. The frequency of consumption can be expressed as an annual measure (see table 5-2).

In some instances, it is possible to refine the estimated frequency of consumption by combining food consumption data with industry information such as annual sales volume or market share information. For example, if the food consumption data report the frequency of consumption of a broad category such as milk, market share data may be used to predict the frequency of consuming particular types of milk. Note that in making this prediction, some assumptions will need to be made. For instance, if $x\%$ of all orange juice sales are for calcium-fortified orange juice, then it may be appropriate to assume that that same percentage applies to consumption. It will also be necessary to consider whether the *amount* of calcium-fortified juice that is consumed is similar across brands of orange juice and across the population.

Assessing Food Intake

Consumption Data Validation

Validation of food intake information from food surveys is a particular problem because there is no absolute standard for estimating the true usual intakes of a free-living person. Five approaches have been taken to validate food surveys, including (1) observation of intake, (2) weighing food before selection and consumption, (3) comparing two approaches of reporting intake, (4) laboratory analysis of duplicate meals or food portions, and (5) biochemical determinations of a physiological variable related to a specific nutrient (Willett, 1990; Cameron, 1988). Studies have been conducted to compare the validity of one type of food survey with another method. Studies comparing estimated food records with weighed portions of foods showed mixed results. In one study, approximately 9% of all food items were omitted in the estimated records. However, in another study, 81% of the respondents underreported foods (Life Science Research Office, 1989). Validity studies of 24-hour recall surveys indicated that reporting errors occur. However, the direction (i.e., under- or over-

TABLE 5-2 Expression of consumption as an annual measure

Number of days annually on which the food is consumed
Number of eating occasions over a year
Annual number of meals
Number of times the food is consumed per year
Number of 100-g portions consumed in a year
Percentage of the population who ate the food in a specific time period (e.g., year)

reporting) and the extent of errors were not consistent from study to study. It is likely that 24-hour recall surveys face underreporting problems similar to those found with food records (Willett, 1990). Validation studies on food frequency surveys also showed mixed results; a study comparing the results of food frequencies with the actual weighed diets of the respondents indicated that several foods were frequently omitted and the frequency of consumption of foods was correctly reported only 51% of the time (Life Science Research Office, 1993).

Laboratory analyses of duplicate meals or food samples have also been used as a validation technique. In one study, duplicate 24-hour food collections were used to validate the use of simultaneous one-day food diaries in a subsample of 24 high school students. A correlation coefficient of 0.75 was observed between sodium values computed from food diaries and laboratory analysis of sodium in duplicate food collections (Willett, 1990).

Nitrogen content of urine has been used to verify protein intake. For example, if protein intake calculated from the reported food intake is in agreement with protein intake calculated from nitrogen excretion, it is assumed that intake of other nutrients is valid (Bingham and Cummings, 1985). The problem with this validating method is that levels of some nutrients in plasma serum and urine are regulated more by physiological mechanisms than by diet. (Willett, 1990).

Reliability and Sources of Error

Reliability, or reproducibility, is the ability of a method to produce the same or similar estimate on two or more different occasions, whether or not the estimate is accurate. For example, the reliability of food consumption survey data for estimating "usual" intake of a population depends somewhat on the number of days of dietary intake data collected for each individual in the population. The number of days of food consumption data required for reliable estimation of population intakes is related to each subject's day-to-day variation in diet (intraindividual variation) and the degree to which subjects differ from each other in their diets (interindividual variation) (Basiotis et al., 1987; Nelson et al., 1989). When intraindividual variation is small relative to interindividual variation, population intakes can be reliably estimated with consumption data from a smaller number of days than should be obtained if both types of variation are large. Intake of contaminants can be reliably estimated with fewer days of data when they are present in many foods that are commonly consumed.

Usual Intakes

While there are challenges associated with sampling and measuring residues in foods, surveying population food consumption patterns presents another set of challenges since diets vary greatly from individual to individual and from day to day. Many factors influence the individual and family choices to acquire and consume foods, including household income, price of foods, personal factors (e.g., age, sex, ethnic group, employment status, education), physiological status (e.g., pregnancy), and environmental factors such as advertising or convenience (Cameron, 1988; Life Science Research Office, 1989).

Intake distributions for many dietary components are skewed to the right. The usual dietary intake of a food is the long-run average daily intake of that food that is unobservable. When long-term patterns of consumption (subchronic and chronic exposures) are of a concern rather than consumption levels on any given day (acute exposure), usual intakes are of interest (Sempos et al., 1985; National Research Council, 1986, as cited in Life Science Research Office, 1989; Carriquiry et al., 1992; Nusser et al., 1993).

Although the 24-hour recall has been the most common method used to collect food intake information, it is the least ideal for estimating usual and longer term average daily food intakes. This is because there are considerable variations in intake between days, and it is usually impossible to identify a representative day. These large variations in day-to-day intake of food within individuals (i.e., intraindividual variation) are often greater than interindividual variation. Ratios of the two, however, also differ among foods and food components; among age, sex, and socioeconomic groups; and within and between dietary intake instruments (Pao and Cypel, 1990, as cited in Federation of American Societies for Experimental Biology, 1993; Life Science Research Office, 1986, 1989; National Research Council, 1986, as cited in Life Science Research Office, 1989).

Also of issue is the number of days for which dietary recalls or records are obtained. It has been recommended that greater restrictions be placed on the interpretation of data obtained for a single day than on data obtained over multiple days. Single-day intake data usually result in a distribution that is flatter and wider than the true distribution of usual intakes of individuals in the population. Thus, the prevalence of high or low intakes is overestimated. One-day intake data for each individual is not sufficient for the estimation of usual food intake distributions because the data do not provide a means for distinguishing the intraindividual (within) from the interindividual (among) variances. Multiple days of intake data could provide a means of reducing the effects of intraindividual variation on estimates of usual food intakes. Overestimation has been reported to increase as the number of days of intakes observed for an individual declines (Nusser et al., 1993; Beaton et al., 1979; National Research Council, 1986, as cited in Life Science Research Office, 1989; Life Science Research Office, 1986, 1989).

It is difficult to accurately estimate chronic dietary exposure because of the general lack of long-term food consumption data. Because of respondent burdens and costs, most surveys using food records or recall methodology can capture only a few days of consumption for the same individual, particularly when extensive details (e.g., food quantity, source, ingredients, and preparation method) are collected. On the other hand, food frequency surveys generally capture information about eating patterns over a longer period of time. However, the information collected is not as detailed as that collected by food recall or records surveys. While data from food frequency questionnaires have been used extensively to assess exposure in epidemiological studies, their utility in quantitative exposure assessment for risk characterization has not been thoroughly explored.

Quantitative dietary exposure assessments for risk characterization have been based mainly on information collected from quantitative food surveys such as the 24-hour recall and food records in the USDA surveys. This separation exemplifies the disconnect between the information needs in risk assessment and the tools/information available from epidemiology. A number of methods have been described to generate usual/long-term intakes from 24-hour recall. Nevertheless, none of these methods exploited the available empirical data from the frequency surveys, even though the complementary nature of the food frequency and quantitative surveys had been previously noted.

Nonusers

Users are individuals who reported consuming foods, and nonusers are those who did not report consumption. Because of the large number of nonusers for foods not consumed by most on a daily basis, consumption distributions can be bimodal. The shape of consumption distribution is derived from a mixture of nonusers, usually assigned intake values of zeros, and users with positive consumption values. Complications usually exist because nonusers are not distinguishable from infrequent consumers who did not consume during the sample period (Nusser et al., 1993). Consumption distributions assuming all nonusers have zero consumption could result in underestimates of consumption. However, distributions based on users only would overestimate consumption.

Food Ingredient and Contaminant Intake Assessment

To evaluate food ingredient or contaminant intakes, three types of data are generally needed: (1) food consumption information, (2) residue concentrations in the foods consumed, and (3) proportion of foods containing the compound being evaluated. Consumption data are described in detail above under food intake assessment. Details on the evaluation of food components, ingredients, and contaminants are provided here. The concentration data may be collected through monitoring programs or from controlled experimental studies. The main purposes of monitoring studies are to catch violations and focus on extremes to deter violations, describe distribution of exposure, estimate averages, define representative values, and determine effects of selected factors on residue/exposure. Examples of contaminant monitoring programs include the USDA's Pesticide Data Program and MARCIS Monitoring Program, the Food and Drug Administration's Enforcement Monitoring Program and Total Diet Studies, and the California Environmental Protection Agency's Food Safety Programs.

Market basket surveys sample foods at the point of purchase. Samples are thus collected close to the point of consumption, and concentrations detected in these samples reflect potential increases or decreases in concentrations resulting from contaminant growth, cross-contamination, or residue dissipation. Typically, samples are collected from supermarkets or terminal distribution centers from several geographical regions to cover for potential regional differences in foods that are locally produced and distributed. Often, when monitoring data or field trial studies are not available, regulatory limits such as maximum residue limits (or tolerances) may be used as a proxy for actual exposure measurements. Tolerances are maximum pesticide residue levels legally permitted in food when the substance is applied according to maximum label conditions.

Proportion of Foods Containing the Compound Being Evaluated

When attempting to estimate the amount of contamination, ingredient, or other exposure associated with a food item, it is unlikely that levels are homogeneous throughout the food supply. Thus, it is necessary to estimate the proportion of the food supply containing levels of the substance. In the case of pesticide residue in foods from intentional use as part of growing a crop, market use data can provide information on market share of the products, frequency of application, and amount of product applied, which in turn can be used to generate better estimates of the distributions of exposure. The calculations can be adjusted by incorporating modifiers to reflect the market share or the frequency of consumption. It may also be necessary to make adjustments to reflect differences in the level of detail in different data sets.

Laboratory analysis of ingredients or contaminants may include many samples with levels below the sensitivity of the analytical method (see figure 5-1). These may be true zeros or may contain minute levels of the ingredient or contaminant, and a number of methods are used to adjust for the limitations of the laboratory tests. One method is to assign a value to all samples (e.g., half the limit of detection) or to assign a value to a percentage of the samples. These

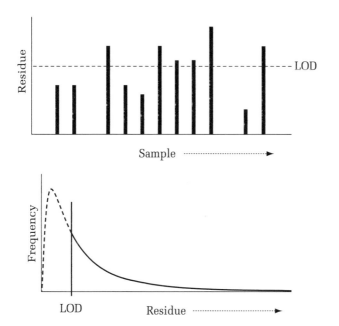

Figure 5-1. Typical environmental data may include censored observations, that is, concentrations below the sensitivity of the analytical method (LOD, limit of detection).

methods may affect the average or median value for a distribution; however, they would have a lesser effect on the upper percentile estimates of exposure.

Another problem frequently encountered is inadequate data for subpopulations with extreme exposures, for example, children and infants. Where data are missing, it may be necessary to utilize a conservative "default" estimate for that parameter. The impact of the value chosen for such defaults should be tested.

Mapping Residue Data to Food Consumption Data

Consumption data collected from surveys typically refer to specific foods such as apple pie or pepperoni pizza; however, exposure data for pesticide residues, chemicals, and other components may be available only for raw agricultural commodities, such as chicken or corn. Thus, recipes and translation factors are needed to convert the amounts reported for foods as consumed into the corresponding raw agricultural commodities. For instance, if a survey participant reported consuming 100 gm of apple pie, an "apple pie recipe" can be applied to translate that intake into the various ingredients (flour, sugar, fat/oil, apples; see figure 5-2).

Adjustment factors needed to translate the consumption amounts of the ingredients (flour, oil, etc.) into their equivalent raw agricultural commodity components are typically derived from USDA Handbook 102 (U.S. Department of Agriculture, 1975) and USDA Commodity Maps (U.S. Department of Agriculture, 1982). Both of these sources provide information on the quantity of processed foods from a unit amount of whole commodity. The USDA Commodity Maps document specifically lists conversion factors (measures of the physical transformation of a commodity from farm gate to processing/consumption) for many foods.

The conversion factor is the ratio of the weight of the commodity in one form to its weight in another form. The factors reflect gains or losses in a commodity. For example, the conversion factor reported for apple juice is 0.774 pounds per pound of fresh apples, indicating that one pound of apples converts to 0.774 pounds of apple juice. If residue data are available only for the whole apple, this conversion factor may be used to determine the potential impact on the pesticide residues if treated whole apples are processed to juice. That is, since 1.3 pounds of apples are needed to produce one pound of apple juice, it is assumed that the pesticide level in the apples would concentrate 1.3 times in the processed juice (1 ÷ 0.774). Conversion information may change over time as a result of the adoption of new technology in both production and processing as well as variation in the physical properties of commodities from one crop year to another. In addition, as new products become available in the market, new conversion factors may be warranted.

Estimating Residue Intake

Exposure to food ingredients or contaminants can be estimated based on the dietary exposure model previously described in equation 1. This model will

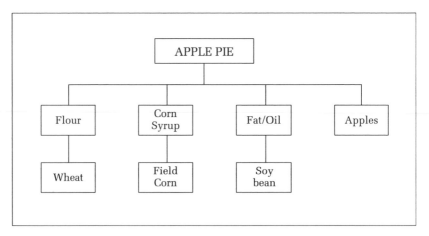

Figure 5-2. The use of recipes to convert foods as eaten into raw agricultural commodities to match the residue data.

need to take into account variations in concentrations of the chemical, variations in food consumption patterns, and variations in the exposed individual's personal characteristics. Personal characteristics, including body weight, cooking methods, and so on, vary not only between individuals but also from day to day or season to season within individuals. Similarly, concentration levels vary depending on when and where they are measured, when and where the chemical was applied, the extent of commercial processing, and so forth. Since pesticide usage may be seasonal, a calendar-based approach to derive the probability distribution of potential exposures is most suitable.

Monte Carlo modeling allows the assessment of major contributing factors to the overall exposure. Sensitivity analyses can be performed to show which factors contribute most to the variability in the exposure distributions and where additional data may be needed to better define the exposure estimates.

Examples of Probabilistic Assessment

Since concentrations in foods and amounts of foods consumed are variable, probabilistic models that combine distributions of concentrations and amounts consumed produce more realistic estimates of intakes than do deterministic methods. Simulation techniques, referred to as "Monte Carlo" methods, combine different permutations of consumption and concentration levels to produce the likelihood and the magnitude of dietary intake levels.

Correlations

Where correlations between data parameters are known to exist, they should be accounted for in the model. Intraindividual correlations include the selection of foods on a given day and on sequential days. There are well-documented correlations between intakes on sequential days. There can also be interindividual correlations. For example, food eaten by individuals in the same household would be correlated. Figure 5-3 shows an example of the correlation of the intake of two foods by the same individual. There are individuals who consume relatively large amounts of apples and individuals who consume large amounts of tomatoes, but no individuals consume large amounts of both tomatoes and apples.

Estimating the Number of Microbiological Organisms in Foods

Similar to the method used in assessing intakes of food ingredients and contaminants, assessing intakes of a food microbial agent requires two types of

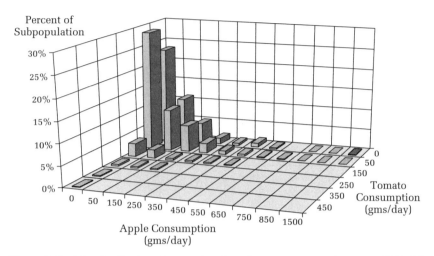

Figure 5-3. Joint distribution of reported apple and tomato consumption among U.S. children 1–6 years of age: 1989–1991 USDA CSFII.

information: food consumption information and expected quantity of the microbial agent in the food consumed. Extensive discussion on evaluating the expected quantity of the microbial agents in foods can be found in chapter 9 on food risk assessment. Food consumption data are described in detail above under food intake assessment.

The results of a food microbial risk assessment can be expressed as probabilities of potential adverse outcomes for an individual, both on a per-serving basis (i.e., number of illnesses per serving) and on an individual basis (i.e., chance of food-borne illness per year), and as population-based risks. These depend on development of food intake metrics such as serving size (in weight), annual number of servings per person, total annual number of servings, or, for example, percentage of the population who are consumers.

In an outbreak investigation, information about food intakes is usually obtained during hypothesis-generating interviews. The objective of hypothesis-generating interviews is to explore all potential sources of infection with a limited number of affected individuals/patients (or their surrogates). For hypothesis-generating interviews to be most informative, efforts are usually made to interview a variety of patients (i.e., with different demographic characteristics). The typical focus of hypothesis-generating interviews is summarized in table 5-3.

In taking the food history, patients (or their surrogates) are asked open-ended questions about foods eaten in their home as well as at restaurants, fast-food establishments, delis, and the homes of friends and family. The purpose of these questions is to identify all possible relevant foods. The result of the open-

TABLE 5-3   Typical focus of hypothesis-generating interviews

Demographic information
Clinical details of the illness with date of onset, duration, and severity of symptoms
Visits to health care providers or hospitals, and laboratory results
A complete food history in the last seven days
Water exposure in the last seven days (e.g., drinking water, exposure to recreational
   waters)
Exposure to other ill persons in the last seven days
Exposure to children in daycare in the last seven days
Exposure to a farm or farm animals in the last seven days
Travel outside the immediate area in the last seven days

ended interview is a list of all foods consumed during a given period. For example, in an investigation of *Yersinia enterocolitica* infections in young children in Belgium, open-ended interviews of the mothers of some of the ill children showed that many gave their children raw pork sausage as a weaning food, providing the first clue as to the source of these infections (Tauxe et al., 1987). Other data typically collected during these interviews are the names and addresses of commercial food-serving establishments, date and time of food consumption, and any unusual observations. To help jog patients' memory, they are often asked to use a calendar or appointment book in providing the food history, focusing on prominent events, weekends, or holidays. Another efficient method is to ask patients to reconstruct each day in the time period of interest, meal by meal.

In addition to the more open-ended questions about exposures, patients may be asked specific questions about consumption of certain food items that have been linked to specific microbiological infections. For example, if *E. coli* O157:H7 infection is involved, patients would be asked whether they have had recent consumption of hamburger/ground beef, lettuce, apple cider, unpasteurized apple juice, or raw alfalfa, all of which have been implicated in other outbreaks.

The commonalities among these patients (as well as other information collected early in the outbreak) provide the basis for the hypotheses about the source of the outbreak. These hypotheses can then be specifically tested in subsequent analytical-epidemiological (and other) studies, whose goals are to assess the relationship between a given exposure and the disease under study. While risk assessment requires quantitative estimates of food intakes, such estimates are not used in the initial descriptive and subsequent analytic epidemiology. As such, refined food intake estimates are neither collected nor estimated in an outbreak investigation. Exposure classification is simply based on whether or not the patient ate the food item of interest during a relevant exposure period. In cases where leftovers of the implicated food or duplicates (food from same supply batches) are available, laboratory analysis could be conducted to definitively determine if the food is the source of the infection. However, even in these cases, quantitative estimates (i.e., colony-forming units) are not usually determined.

Summary reports of food-borne disease outbreaks often lack information about the degree of contamination in the implicated food and the amount of the implicated food item consumed by members of the exposed population (Jones et al., 2004). Due to the lack of emphasis on more robust exposure estimates, results of outbreak investigations have had limited utility in risk assessment, which provides the basis for regulatory decision. This disconnect between the need of quantitative exposure for risk assessment and lack thereof in epidemiology has been previously noted (Matanoski, 1988). To bridge this gap, an intensive investigation questionnaire template that contains a list of questions to be asked of exposed people in an outbreak investigation has been developed by Jones et al. (2004). In the future, increasing focus on quantifying food intake/exposure information in outbreak investigations not only will enhance the conclusions from these investigations but also will help reduce the existing large uncertainties in food microbial risk assessment (i.e., the dose response).

References

Australia New Zealand Food Authority. 1997. Dietary modeling: principles and procedures. Author.

Basiotis, P.P., S.O. Welsh, J. Cronin, J.L. Kelsay, and W. Mertz. 1987. Number of days of food intake records required to estimate individual and group nutrient intakes with defined confidence. J. Nutr. 117:1638–1641.

Beaton, G.H., J. Milner, P. Corey, V. McGuire, M. Cousins, E. Stewart, E. de Ramos, D. Hewitt, P.V. Grambsch, N. Kassim, and J.A. Little. 1979. Sources of variance in 24-hour dietary recall data: implications for nutrition study design and interpretation. Am. J. Clin. Nutr. 32: 2546–2559.

Bingham, S., and J.H. Cummings. 1985. Urine nitrogen as an independent validatory measure of dietary intake: a study of nitrogen balance in individuals consuming their normal diet. Am. J. Clin. Nutr. 42:1276–1289.

Cameron, M.E., and W.A. Van Staveren, eds. 1988. Manual on methodology for food consumption studies. Oxford, U.K.: Oxford University Press.

Carriquiry, A.L., H. Jensen, K.W. Dodd, S.M. Nusser, L.G. Borred, and W.A. Fuller. 1992. Estimating usual intake distributions. Journal Paper No. J-14654, Project No. 2806. Ames: Iowa Agriculture and Home Economics Experiment Station.

Fujita, M., and K. Morikawa. (1992). Regional differences in dietary intake of environmental pollutants in Japan. J. Exp. Anal. Envirn. Epid. 2(2):177–193.

Hill, R.H., S.L. Head, S. Baker, M. Gregg, D.B. Shealy, S.L. Bailey, C.V. Williams, E.J. Sampson, and L.L. Sampson. 1995. Pesticide residues in the urine of adults living in the United States: reference range concentrations. Environ. Res. 71(2):99–108.

Jones, R.C., S.I. Gerber, P.S. Diaz, L.L. Williams, S.B. Dennis, E.S. Parish, and W.S. Paul. 2004. Intensive investigation of bacterial food-borne disease outbreaks: proposed guidelines and tools for the collection of dose-response data by local health departments. J. Food Prot. 67(3):616–623.

Life Sciences Research Office. 1986. Guidelines for use of dietary intake data. Bethesda, MD: Federation of American Societies for Experimental Biology.

Life Science Research Office. 1988. Estimation of exposure to substances in the food supply. Bethesda, MD: Federation of American Societies for Experimental Biology.

Life Science Research Office. 1989. Nutrition monitoring in the United States, an update report on nutrition monitoring. DHHS Publication No. (PHS) 89–1255.

Life Science Research Office. 1993. NHEXAS dietary monitoring options. Bethesda, MD: Federation of American Societies for Experimental Biology.

Liu, K., J. Stamler, A. Dyer, J. McKeever, and P. McKeever. 1978. Statistical methods to assess and minimize the role of intra-individual variability in obscuring the relationship between dietary lipids and serum cholesterol. J. Chron. Dis. 31:399–418.

Matanoski, G.M. 1988. Issues in the measurement of exposure. Chapter 9 in Epidemiology and health risk assessment (Gordis, L., ed.). Oxford, U.K.: Oxford University Press.

Natural Resource Defense Concil (NRDC). Intolerable Risk: Pesticides in Our Children's Food. Feb 27, 1989.

Nelson, M., A.E. Black, J.A. Morris, and T.J. Cole. 1989. Between- and within-subject variation in nutrient intake from infancy to old age: estimating the number of days required to rank dietary intakes with desired precision. Am. J. Clin. Nutr. 50:155–167.

Nusser, S.M., Carriquiry, A.L., and Fuller, W.A. 1993. A semiparametric transformation approach to estimating usual daily intake distributions. Ames: Iowa State University.

Petersen, B., and L. Barraj. 1996. Assessing the intake of contaminants and nutrients: a review of methods. J. Food Comp. Anal. 9:243–254.

Petersen, B., and J. Douglass. 1994. Use of food-intake surveys to estimate exposure to non-nutrients. Am. J. Clin. Nutrit. 59(suppl.):2403–2433.

Rees, N.M.A., and D.R. Tennant. (1993). Estimating consumer intakes of food chemical contaminants. In Safety of Chemicals in Food (David Watson, Ed.). Chichester, U.K.: Ellis Horwood

Scientific Committee on Foods Intake and Exposure Working Group. 1994. Summaries of food consumption databases in the European Union. CS/Int/Gen2 (European Commission). Brussels: Author.

Sempos, C.T., N.E. Johnson, E.L. Smith, and C. Gilligan. 1985. Effects of intra-individual and inter-individual variation in repeated dietary records. Am. J. Epidemiol. 121:120–130.

Tauxe, R.V., G. Walters, V. Goossen, R. VanNoyer, J. Vandepitte, S.M. Martin, et al. 1987. Yersinia enterocolitica infections and pork: the missing link. Lancet 5:1129–1132.

Trichopoulou, A., and P. Lagiou, eds. 1997. Methodology for the exploitation of HBS food data and results on food availability in 5 European countries. Data Food Networking.

U.S. Department of Agriculture. 1975. Food yields summarized by different stages of preparation. Agriculture Handbook No. 102. Author.

U.S. Department of Agriculture. 1999. Continuing survey of food intakes by individuals. Online. ARS Food Surveys Research Group, available on the "Products and services" page at http://www.ars.usda.gov/Services/docs.htm?docid=7825 (accessed 11/07/06).

Waldman, J. M., P.J Lioy, A. Greenberg, and J.P. Butler. (1991). Analysis of human exposure to benzo(a)pyrene via inhalation and food ingestion in the total human environmental exposure study (THEES). J. Exp. Anal. Envirn. Epid. 1(2):193–225.

Willett, W. (1990). Nutritional epidemiology. Oxford, U.K.: Oxford University Press.

6

MANAGING A FOOD-BORNE OUTBREAK

Tamar Lasky

The classic food-borne outbreak occurs at a small church picnic, where a well-meaning individual leaves potato salad out in warm temperatures or someone who just came in from feeding the cows begins to slice the ham without first washing his or her hands. Fifteen minutes or one hour or several hours after the picnic (depending on the pathogen), a number of attendees are suffering from nausea or diarrhea, and in a small community, word of mouth quickly establishes that an outbreak has taken place. The local or state health department then comes by with a questionnaire, asks everyone who attended the picnic to list the foods they ate, and makes a quick tabulation of attack rates by food to identify the vehicle of transmission. The health officials collect stool, vomit, and blood samples and compare these with food samples as a means of identifying the pathogen and confirming the presence of the pathogen in the foods. After the church supper or picnic, all remaining food is thrown out, and there the outbreak would end.

Such outbreaks still occur and still make the news. On July 13, 2002, the *Boston Globe* reported, "Hospital Flooded with Food Poisoning Cases after Church Supper." About 200 people attended the church supper in Newport, Maine, and at least 23 were hospitalized at the closest hospital, Sebasticook Valley Hospital. The church supper menu included ham, mashed potatoes, scalloped onions, cranberry salad, rolls, pies, cold drinks, coffee, and tea. At the time of the report, the pathogen and vehicle had not been identified (Associated Press 2002).

Recognizing a Food-Borne Outbreak

The church supper outbreak scenario is one of the simplest to recognize—people in a relatively small group, many of whom know each other well, eat a limited menu and become sick shortly after the meal. The food is consumed or thrown away, the outbreak runs its course, and concern does not spread beyond the circle of people who were directly affected. Public health officials continuously warn people to avoid leaving foods at room temperatures at picnics and suppers and to use safe food-handling practices, and such outbreaks continue to occur because the advice is disregarded. While troublesome and inconvenient, these types of outbreaks do not seem to cause a great deal of worry in the general public, nor do they stop people from holding or attending church suppers or picnics.

Beyond the church supper, outbreaks can take on endless permutations, occurring in restaurants, school lunch programs, hospitals, and other food service settings, resulting from contamination and/or mishandling at the farm, the processing plant, the manufacturer, or the final point of preparation. When contamination occurs close to the point of consumption and in the home, relatively few people are affected, and the outbreak is limited by the size of the household. Exposures through food may be indistinguishable from general exposures that occur between household members sharing the same space, bathrooms, and sleeping quarters. If, however, contamination of household food precedes a social function, a true food-borne outbreak can occur and be recognized. Outbreaks after family parties, weddings, or family-hosted community meetings such as Girl Scouts or PTA continue to occur. Carelessness in home food preparation can lead to an outbreak if enough people outside of the household are exposed to the food, but most of the time, contamination of food in the home is limited in its effects to the household members. Food-borne illnesses occurring in the same household are generally not considered to be outbreaks, even though they are counted in surveillance of total cases of food-borne illness.

In the past, outbreaks were often defined as epidemics or as an increased incidence of disease over and above some background level. The rise in the occurrence of a disease, symptom, syndrome, or cause of death would indicate a change in exposure levels, virulence, susceptibilities, rates of transmission, or other factors and would warrant an epidemiologic investigation. In all fields of epidemiology, recognition of this early change in incidence is key to understanding the "outbreak"—whether it is chronic and spread over decades, as in the increase in lung cancer rates following the rise of smoking, or whether it is acute and occurs in a few days following contamination at a restaurant. A standard operating definition of a food-borne disease outbreak is "the occurrence of two or more cases of the same clinical illness among people from different households resulting from the ingestion of the same food or meal" (International Association of Milk, Food, and Environmental Sanitarians, Inc. 1999). This definition rules out single cases of food-borne illness as well as multiple cases occurring within the same household.

Investigating Food-Borne Outbreaks

Local or state health departments are often the first to receive reports of a food-borne outbreak—the reports might come directly from the public or from restaurants, schools, organizers of a church picnic, daycare centers, or other groups receiving complaints from people who think they became ill as a result of food consumed at that particular organization. Reports may also come from practitioners recognizing an unusual case or an unusual number of cases. There is no set pattern for recognizing these initial cases because they occur before the outbreak is formally recognized. Sometimes it takes only two or three cases to alert a local or state health department that an outbreak has occurred—this depends on the background rate and the size of the group affected. For example, three cases occurring in a school in a one- or two-day period is different than three cases occurring throughout a city over a week—the first situation is easier to recognize as a potential outbreak, and the second situation may or may not be an outbreak with a common source.

Once an outbreak is recognized and publicized in the media, an increase in case reports generally occurs. People report cases they might not have reported had they not heard the media reports. After hearing descriptions of the outbreak in the news, people with similar symptoms may feel more inclined to report their symptoms, and people who suspect that they have been exposed (e.g., by having eaten at the suspected restaurant) may be more alert to their own symptoms. Similarly, practitioners, school nurses, and other health care providers may be encouraged to report cases, collect samples, and request laboratory tests, and people may be more likely to seek medical care.

As case reports come into various government agencies and an outbreak is recognized, the first step is simultaneously to organize an investigational team and to agree on which agency has the lead in handling the investigation. Outbreaks may be recognized at the local, state, or federal level and at different agencies within each level, for example, the state health or agriculture departments or the federal agencies at the U.S. Department of Health and Human Services (Centers for Disease Control and Prevention [CDC] and Food and

Drug Administration [FDA]) and at the U.S. Department of Agriculture (Food Safety and Inspection Service [FSIS]).

One principle determining who takes the lead is that the lowest level of government takes the lead until the outbreak crosses municipal or state boundaries, at which point a higher level must coordinate the investigation. Another principle is that the agency that first recognizes the outbreak continues to lead the investigation. Thus, if complaints coming to an FDA or FSIS consumer hotline lead to an investigation, these agencies might continue to lead the outbreak investigation. As the outbreak investigation proceeds and potential vehicles, agents, and points along the farm-to-table continuum are identified, the necessary regulatory bodies are brought in, and this may include groups regulating labor, manufacturing, transportation, and other interests.

The food-borne outbreak investigation is essentially a scientific study that takes place in an extremely public and political atmosphere, compressed in a relatively short period of time. The media expect daily or hourly updates, as do politicians in affected constituencies and any stakeholders affected by the outbreak (e.g., restaurant workers, retail outlets, manufacturers, other consumers). This context greatly changes the nature of the scientific investigation, and while the focus of this chapter is on the scientific issues, an outbreak investigator would be naive to think that the investigation can proceed without careful attention to the public, media, and political concerns. Those leading outbreak investigations must be prepared to provide succinct summaries at very short notice and in laymen's language and to provide guidance, suggestions, and reassurance even when the data have not yet been collected or analyzed. It is paradoxical, and a touch unreasonable, but it is the nature of the game.

Another pressure that outbreak investigators must work under is the awareness that various types of litigation might follow the conclusion of the outbreak; for example, consumers might sue producers or restaurateurs, or manufacturers might protest and litigate regulatory actions or even sue the media. The patients who became ill during the outbreak need to have medical privacy; at the same time, the public and politicians want to know every detail about every case. Furthermore, each level of government has different constraints on information that can be shared with other agencies, other levels of government, and the public.

The leader of an outbreak investigation needs to follow the guidelines and practices of his or her agency or organization. If the outbreak investigation is being conducted within a private organization such as a school, hospital, or university, it still needs to meet the requirements of its locality. Those who have the responsibility of leading an outbreak investigation will be aware of the relevant guidelines of their organization, and members of the team need to be aware that the leaders are working under a set of specific guidelines.

Most state health departments now have websites outlining their practices and procedures. For example, the Oregon Department of Human Services and the Massachusetts Department of Public Health both have websites that provide investigative guidelines, questionnaire templates and instruction, instructions for collection of stool specimens, and forms for requesting virology/immunology tests, bacteriology/parasitology tests, and mycobacteriology tests. Other organizations such as the International Association of Milk, Food and Environmental Sanitarians, Inc. and the CDC also provide guidelines, flow charts, data collection forms, and other tools for outbreak investigation. Each epidemiologist investigating an outbreak will need to use the approach adopted by his or her organization. Interestingly enough, no one has summarized the different guidelines to describe commonalities or contradictions, and no one has systematically compared approaches to find which approach works best in which situation.

Because the specific tools and details vary by organization, this chapter takes a broad, conceptual approach to an outbreak investigation and attempts to relate this to work done by epidemiologists in other types of investigations. Epidemiological investigations go through four general phases: (1) describing the disease and counting cases, (2) formulating testable hypotheses, (3) designing and conducting a study to test hypotheses, and (4) statistical analysis of study results. In an outbreak investigation all four phases may be so compressed in time that it is difficult to distinguish the phases and even maintain awareness of the distinct phases—the tasks of describing cases, forming hypotheses, designing the study, and analyzing results might take place in a matter of days and might go through several quick iterations, blurring the distinction between phases. Nonetheless, it is useful to be aware of each phase.

Describing Cases and Exposures

In an outbreak investigation, a case definition can be a highly specific set of symptoms, a distinctive pulsed-field gel electrophoresis (PFGE) pattern, or any combination of symptoms and laboratory findings. Case definitions sometimes change over an outbreak investigation; the first three patients might report diarrhea only, while the fourth patient also reports vomiting. The investigators need to decide if the fourth case belongs with the first three cases, is a variant of the same disease, or is a separate condition altogether. Decisions about inclusion or exclusion of cases in an outbreak investigation can be highly fluid, changing daily with acquisition of new information, changing with hypotheses about the disease, and in turn, affecting data analyses. For example, if an outbreak takes place at a daycare center, investigators might decide to exclude cases who do not attend the daycare center and then might reverse that decision upon learning that one case occurred in a school group that visited the daycare center for a holiday celebration. Fluctuation in the case count and case definition is almost inevitable and leads to conflicting conclusions from data analysis. Outbreak cases are subject to both types of misclassification: undercounting and overcounting. Some cases do not come to the attention of the outbreak investigators (e.g., a person who eats at a restaurant and then flies overseas the following day), and some cases are counted in the disease group who might have acquired their illness through another source. While the haste of an outbreak investigation makes this unavoidable, it would be interesting to review some outbreak investigations and analyze ways in which the case definitions might have affected the study results.

Government health departments generally have the authority to conduct interviews with persons who have become ill in a food-borne outbreak, and it is not necessary to prepare lengthy study protocols or receive approval for questionnaires from outside the responsible department, for example, from an institutional review board. Indeed, as mentioned above, most health departments have questionnaires at the ready and a sequence of questions to ask people sickened in an outbreak (box 6-1). Questions include identifying information such as name, address, telephone number; demographics such as age, sex, and occupation; symptoms such as nausea, vomiting, diarrhea, fever, abdominal cramps, muscle aches, chills, fatigue, and bloody diarrhea; date and time of symptoms; food and drink consumption history for at least 72 hours before illness onset; and contact information. Stool samples are collected where possible, and other specimens are collected as needed.

In addition to standard laboratory testing to identify the pathogen species, sophisticated methods such as PFGE can provide more detailed information about subtypes and help distinguish cases that are truly part of the same outbreak. When cases do not have a readily apparent factor in common (e.g., attendance at the same event or eating at the same restaurant), PFGE typing can help group the cases by subtype (Sails et al. 2003). It can also be used to confirm the link between a source and the outbreak victims, as in the investigation of infections of *Campylobacter jejuni* in Kansas, where isolates from a sick cafeteria worker showed the same PFGE pattern as did the isolates from the eight people who became sick after eating at the cafeteria (Olsen et al. 2001).

Because of the time urgency, exposure investigations begin as quickly as possible. Without even conducting a formal analysis, the investigators may conclude that a specific meal, restaurant, or event was the source of the contamination. In such situations, food samples from the meal, restaurant, or event should be taken as soon as possible to confirm hypotheses about the vehicle that was contaminated. Upon hearing that three people eating at a church supper were later ill, the investigator would probably conclude that something at the church supper caused the illness—case finding, hypothesis formation, and hypothesis testing might occur within a two- or three-day period.

BOX 6-1

The CDC provides a standardized questionnaire as an example for those investigating a food-borne outbreak. It is an adaptation of a questionnaire developed by the Minnesota Department of Health. Two sections are reprinted below: part II, which includes questions about clinical symptoms, and the appendix, which asks for a food consumption history.

Part II. Clinical information

Which did you experience <u>first</u>: • vomit   • diarrhea
Date of onset of vomit or diarrhea (whichever occurred first): ____ / ____ / ____

Onset time: *Circle closest hour. For onset times after midnight, double-check the onset day/date!*

1 am	7 am	13–1 pm	19–7 pm
2	8	14–2	20–8
3	9	15–3	21–9
4	10	16–4	22–10
5	11	17–5	23–11
6 am	12 noon	18–6 pm	24–12 midnight

Are you still experiencing vomit or diarrhea?   Y   N
Date of last day of illness with vomit or diarrhea: ____ / ____ / ____
Time of last episode of vomit or diarrhea: ____:____ AM PM

Read questions exactly as written below. Circle Y for "yes," N for "no" and DK for "don't know, can't remember, not sure" etc.
Did you have:

Nausea	Y	N	DK
Vomiting	Y	N	DK
Diarrhea	Y	N	DK

If yes:
Maximum number of stools in a 24-hour period: _____

Bloody diarrhea	Y	N	DK
Abdominal cramps	Y	N	DK
Fever	Y	N	DK
Chills	Y	N	DK
Headache	Y	N	DK
Body aches	Y	N	DK
Fatigue	Y	N	DK
Constipation	Y	N	DK
Other:	Y	N	DK

(continued)

Appendix: Specific food consumption history

Please indicate for each of the food items listed below whether you definitively ate it, maybe ate it, definitively did not eat it, and whether it was
cooked or uncooked, during the seven days before you became ill. The time
period we are talking about is
from _____, ___/___/___ to _____, ___/___/___
[The form has places for information about preparation, brands, store, date
of purchase, and date eaten.]

Dairy
Milk
Buttermilk
Sour cream
Cottage cheese
Cheese
 a. shredded
 b. processed sliced
 c. block
 d. string
 e. curds
Ice cream
Frozen dessert
Yogurt
Meat, poultry
Chicken
Turkey
Hamburger
Hamburger as ingredient
Other beef
Pork
Lamb
Sausage
Fish
Shellfish
Other meat/poultry/fish
Any egg

Fresh Fruits (not canned)
Oranges
Other citrus
Pears
Apples

(continued)

BOX 6-1 (*continued*)

Other tree fruit
Strawberries
Other berries
Grapes
Bananas
Mangoes
Cantaloupe
Watermelon
Other melon
Exotic fruit (specify)

Vegetables (fresh)
Prepackaged salad
Lettuce
  Iceberg
  Red leaf lettuce
  Romaine lettuce
  Mesclun greens
Spinach
Cabbage
Tomatoes
Cucumbers
Peppers
Asparagus
Celery
Carrots
Radishes
Pea pods
Egg plants, squash
Onions
  Green
  Other (white, Spanish)
Broccoli
Fresh herbs
Mushrooms
Cilantro
Sprouts (e.g., on sandwich)
  Alfalfa sprouts
  Bean sprouts
Peanut butter

(*continued*)

Salsa

Dips

Salads

Green (tossed)

Caesar salad

Fruit salad

Pasta salad

Potato salad

Cole slaw

Other Salad

Beverages

Apple juice or cider

Orange juice

Other fruit juice

Iced tea

Special teas, herbal drinks

Source: Centers for Disease Control and Prevention, http://www.cdc.gov/ foodborneoutbreaks/standard_ques.htm.

The investigating team should be able to compile descriptive statistics about the cases, for example, range and mean ages, percentages of males and females, percentages with each symptom, onset of symptoms by hour, day or week (as applicable), and proportion of cases hospitalized or dying.

Outbreak Curve

One of the simplest tools available in an outbreak investigation is a graph plotting the onset of symptoms in the case group by hours, days, or weeks, depending on the illness and the information available. The epidemic curve describes the pattern of transmission. A tight curve with a steep peak suggests a common point of exposure. A peak followed by subsequent lesser peaks may suggest secondary transmission from the first case group or reintroduction of the contaminated food. Several examples of epidemic curves are provided in the case studies at the end of this chapter. The epidemic curve can also be used to estimate the time from exposure to onset of illness, and this information can be used in several ways. When a group of people become sick following a specific meal, such as the church supper, time of onset helps the investigators focus on contaminants that act within the time frame and often leads quickly to the contaminated food item. When the meal has not been identified, and a pathogen has been identified, time of onset can help investigators narrow down the meals that might have provided the opportunity for illness, because different pathogens and diseases follow different sequences following exposure. Some pathogens produce toxins that act within hours, while other pathogens take one to three days or even weeks to infect the person and cause illness.

Developing Hypotheses

In long-term epidemiologic studies, particularly in chronic disease epidemiology, a hypothesis is formally stated a priori. The study design is guided by the requirements of testing the stated hypothesis, and the study findings are interpreted in the context of the study hypothesis. Because research encounters unexpected findings—patient characteristics may differ from what was expected, a treatment may have unanticipated benefits or side effects, a new scientific finding may change the research concerns—many research reports go beyond that of testing and reporting on the tests of the a priori hypothesis.

In an outbreak development and modification of hypotheses may take place rapidly, over a period of hours, and much of the process may be confined to oral conversations in meetings or conference calls. When a health official first receives reports, initial hypotheses immediately come to mind—it was something they ate in the school cafeteria, it was food prepared for the restaurant chain, or produce from farm A was contaminated by the water. Early information generally suggests a limited outbreak with immediate causes, while later information may widen the scope of the outbreak and the investigation.

Study Design for Outbreaks

Older textbooks such as the original edition of A. M. Lilienfeld's *Foundations of Epidemiology* (Oxford University Press, 1976) suggest analyzing data from a food-borne outbreak as a reconstructed cohort. The individuals attending the church supper (or other such event) are members of the cohort. The foods served at the supper are the potential exposures. Persons eating the food item are considered exposed, and persons who did not eat the food item are considered nonexposed. Attack rates are calculated as the number of ill persons divided by the number exposed or unexposed, and relative attack rates compare the attack rate in the exposed to that in the unexposed. The analysis is repeated for each food item (exposure), and the highest relative attack rates suggest the food items that are associated with illness.

The reconstructed cohort approach works best when one strongly suspects a common source (e.g., church supper) and when one can identify all or almost all members of the cohort (attendees at the church supper). In many other situations, one begins with much less information. Case–control approaches help an investigator find some common points of exposure if it is not readily obvious, perhaps a specific restaurant or a food item contaminated at the point of distribution. Selection of controls is critical and is shaped by hypotheses concerning the source of exposure (Lasky and Stolley 1994). For example, if one suspects a specific restaurant, one might select controls who ate at the restaurant in the same period as the cases and who did not become sick; this would allow comparison of foods eaten by the cases and controls. If one does not yet know that a restaurant was the point of exposure, controls might be selected from the neighborhood, through random-digit dialing, or by some other method. Over the past decades, outbreak investigators have increasingly used the case–control method—sometimes appropriately and sometimes without sufficient thought to the complexities of the case–control method. Results of a case–control study are highly influenced by conceptual decisions in case definition and control selection, greatly affecting the odds ratio and potentially introducing biases and/ or spurious results. These methodologic issues have not been explored as they apply to outbreak investigations but have been thoroughly reviewed with respect to cancer epidemiology. The case–control study design has also been applied to the study of aggregate groups of cases that are not part of single outbreak. This particular application is discussed further in chapter 8.

Statistical Analysis

When the hypotheses point to a finite group of consumers (e.g., attendees at a wedding, passengers on a ship, residents of a nursing home), one usually reconstructs the cohort, identifies the foods served, and interviews each member of the cohort to determine which individuals consumed which foods. Attack rates in the exposed are calculated by dividing the number of people who ate the item and became sick by the total number who ate the suspected food item. Attack rates in the unexposed are calculated analogously; the number of people who did not eat the item and became sick is divided by the number of people who did not eat the item. The two attack rates are then compared by dividing the attack rate in the people who ate the food item (exposed) by the attack rates in the people who did not eat the food item (unexposed) to produce the relative risk of disease associated with the specific food item (see box 6-2). The 95% confidence interval is then calculated. Similar calculations are performed for each food item. The relative risk indicates the strength of association between the food item and the disease, and the 95% confidence interval describes the range within which 95% of study results would fall if the study were repeated 100 times. If the 95% confidence interval does not include 1, it suggests that the observed difference between the attack rates in the exposed and unexposed is not explained by chance alone.

Case Studies

There is no way to convey the diversity of outbreak scenarios without reviewing a few examples. Six outbreaks are described below. They are not a ran-

---

BOX 6-2 Calculations of food specific attack rates, relative risks, and 95% confidence intervals

$$\text{Attack rate in exposed} = \frac{\text{Number of people who ate the food item and became sick}}{\text{Total number of people who ate the food item}}$$

$$\text{Attack rate in unexposed} = \frac{\text{Number of people who did not eat the food item and became sick}}{\text{Total number of people who did not eat the food item}}$$

$$\text{Relative risk (RR)} = \frac{\text{Attack rate in exposed}}{\text{Attack rate in unexposed}}$$

$$\text{95\% confidence interval for RR} = (RR)\exp\left[\pm 1.96\sqrt{\text{Variance (ln RR)}}\right]$$

---

dom sample of outbreaks, and they do not demonstrate the full range of variation observed in different outbreaks. They do demonstrate that apparently unique events—exceptions to the rule—are almost the rule. A public health official needs to be prepared to manage a "typical" outbreak, but even more important, a public health official needs to be prepared to manage an outbreak that is unlike previous outbreaks. They occur often, and they may have widespread public health impact, affecting many individuals and businesses and even crossing international boundaries. The six outbreaks described here include outbreaks caused by bacterial, parasitical, viral, and chemical contamination, and an outbreak where more than one pathogen was present. The outbreaks include contamination at the farm, in food preparation, by ill food handlers, and two that appear to result from intentional contamination.

Case Study 1: Viral Contamination of Produce— Hepatitis A at a Restaurant

Hepatitis A is a viral infection of the liver acquired through oral–fecal transmission, and it has an average incubation time of 30 days. By the time symptoms lead the patient to seek medical care, and liver infection is evident, the patient will not necessarily connect his or her illness with any particular food or meal eaten in the previous month. In early November 2003, a clinician reported a case of hepatitis A to the Pennsylvania Department of Health and noted that 10 other cases of hepatitis had been treated recently in a local emergency department (Centers for Disease Control and Prevention 2003). This appears to be the report that alerted public health officials to the possibility of a hepatitis A outbreak—it could have happened a few days earlier or later, but it is a key event in recognizing an outbreak.

The health department searched its records and identified a recently reported case in the same community, with onset several days earlier. These events are described in their Health Alert #61 from November 3, 2003 (see box 6-3). In addition to providing information about events at the moment, they solicit information about other cases and mention that the corporate office had voluntarily closed the restaurant suspected of serving the contaminated food. Two days later, the health department recommended that patrons who had eaten at the restaurant between October 22 and November 2 should receive injections of immune globulin, and also be alert to symptoms of hepatitis A. People who had eaten at the restaurant earlier than October 22 would be outside the 14 day period within which immune globulin injections would be effective. Thus, intervention in the form of recommendations, closure of the restaurant, and immune globulin injections took place as the investigation developed. This is in complete contrast to other types of epidemiologic studies where we await data, analysis, and discussions before implementing efforts to prevent illness. An outbreak investigation is a simultaneous effort to prevent further illness and to uncover the cause of the outbreak. It is also interesting to note that prevention and control of the acute outbreak might be highly successful and immediate, but that the scientific inquiry into causes may lag far behind.

The outbreak investigation grew, and by November 25, 2003, 605 cases of hepatitis A had been reported (including three deaths), all of whom had eaten at the same restaurant in suburban Pittsburgh during the same period in October. Figure 6-1 illustrates the distribution of disease onset dates relative to dates of exposure (eating at the restaurant); the separation in distributions is consistent with the incubation time for hepatitis A.

The outbreak was eventually linked to green onions (scallions) used in the salsa. Although food workers were also ill, investigators did not think that the workers had introduced the contamination because of the timing of their illnesses. Investigators began looking for similar strains associated with other outbreaks, and considered hypotheses suggesting a source of contamination in Mexico, where the scallions were grown. At the time of this writing, the source of contamination had not been determined, and while the outbreak associated with that specific restaurant has ended, the cause of the outbreak is not yet known.

BOX 6-3 Health Alert Network 2003

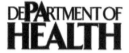

DEPARTMENT OF HEALTH

PENNSYLVANIA DEPARTMENT OF HEALTH HEALTH ALERT #61

To: Health Alert Network
From: Calvin B. Johnson, M.D., M.P.H. Secretary of Health
Date: November 3, 2003
Subject: **Large Outbreak of Restaurant-Associated Hepatitis A**

This transmission is a "Health Alert," conveys the highest level of importance; Warrants immediate action or attention.

HOSPITALS: PLEASE SHARE THIS WITH ALL MEDICAL, INFECTION CONTROL, NURSING, LABORATORY, RADIOLOGY & PHARMACY STAFF IN YOUR HOSPITAL

LOCAL HEALTH JURISDICTIONS: PLEASE DISTRIBUTE AS APPROPRIATE

PROFESSIONAL HEALTH ORGANIZATIONS: PLEASE DISTRIBUTE TO YOUR MEMBERSHIP AS APPROPRIATE

EMS COUNCILS: PLEASE DISTRIBUTE AS APPROPRIATE

Date of Outbreak/Emergency: October 2003

Description of Outbreak/Emergency:

The Pennsylvania Department of Health (PADOH) is investigating an outbreak of hepatitis A among patrons and staff of a Chi-Chi's restaurant in the Beaver Valley Mall in Monaca.

An alert clinician contacted PADOH on Saturday (November 1) to report an IgM-positive hepatitis A case and noted that as many as 10 other cases of hepatitis had been seen recently in a local emergency department. Over the next 36 hours, additional probable cases were identified based on symptoms, and seven other IgM-positive cases were reported. Several adults were admitted to the hospital with extremely high transaminases. Onsets were all in the last week of October.

Review of laboratory results in Pennsylvania's National Electronic Disease Surveillance System (NEDSS) identified one recently reported case of hepatitis A in the same community with onset October 23.

(continued)

All but one community case of hepatitis A interviewed so far had a single common risk factor, eating at the Beaver Valley Mall Chi Chi's restaurant in early October.

It was further learned that at least 10 employees of the restaurant (out of 50 total) were absent from work due to illness in the past week. Interviews with five determined that all five had multiple symptoms consistent with prodromal hepatitis A, also with onsets in the last week of October. Interviews with 13 supposedly well workers found an additional three with possible hepatitis A. Employees routinely eat the same food as patrons. Additional data collection is in progress.

The cluster of onsets in late October among both patrons and employees, and the dates that ill patrons reported eating at the restaurant, are all consistent with exposure during the first few days of October. No single food item has been implicated, and one hypothesis is that an ill food worker inadvertently contaminated multiple food items during preparation or serving.

Description of Action(s) Taken/Planned:

The Department of Agriculture sent an inspector to the restaurant on Saturday afternoon November 1; the inspector found no sanitary violations and emphasized strict hygiene and that all food workers must wear gloves pending further directions from the Department of Health. The restaurant corporate office has voluntarily closed the facility.

A state health center clinic is being arranged to administer immune serum globulin (ISG) to well restaurant workers. A press release that includes the address of the clinic will be released shortly.

Other persons who should consider receiving ISG include:

- Patrons who ate at the restaurant in the previous 14 days (with this large number of ill workers, there is a high risk of additional transmission among recent patrons). It is estimated that the restaurant had 3,400 patrons in the second half of October. Because so many different food items at this restaurant may have bare-hand contact during preparation or serving, including chips and nachos, most patrons can be considered eligible for ISG if they present within 14 days after eating at the Beaver Valley Mall Chi-Chi's.
- Household contacts of any patrons who ate at the restaurant in early October and are ill now with symptoms suggesting hepatitis A (but may not have previously presented for medical care). It is possible that hundreds of persons who ate at the restaurant in early October are now ill or about

(continued)

BOX 6-3 (continued)

to become ill. The incubation period for hepatitis A ranges from two weeks to two months but typically is around 28 days.
- Household contacts of employees already ill with probable hepatitis A

It is anticipated that a large number of people may seek ISG as a result of the press release to be issued shortly. Another goal of the press release is sharing knowledge with the community of the mechanism of hepatitis A transmission, to help reduce additional cases by promoting appropriate hygiene by ill persons.

PADOH advises clinicians to:

- Ask patients presenting with symptoms consistent with hepatitis A whether they dined in the implicated restaurant, or any other restaurant, during the month prior to symptom onset.
- When choosing to test for hepatitis A, order **IgM** antibody testing **specifically**; otherwise some laboratories will test for the presence of total Ig only (which by itself is not useful for making the diagnosis of acute infection).
- Hepatitis A infection is a reportable disease in PA. Prompt notification of your local or state health department will speed termination of the

---

Case Study 2: *E. coli* O157:H7 and Alfalfa Seeds

Escherichia coli O157:H7 is excreted in the feces of cattle and is thus often associated with contaminated meat products; however, cattle manure can contaminate water or the fields where it is used as fertilizer and may contaminate produce. It was first recognized in 1982 and is associated with bloody and nonbloody diarrhea and hemolytic uremic syndrome, a leading cause of kidney failure in children in the United States. Cases of infection with *E. coli* O157:H7 are monitored closely by health departments, and in June and July 1997, two state health departments (Michigan and Virginia) independently investigated outbreaks of *E. coli* O157:H7 (Breuer et al. 2001). Both states sent isolates to the CDC for PFGE subtyping. All isolates had indistinguishable PFGE patterns with restriction enzymes XbaI and BlnI. PFGE typing led to identification of cases from other states, broadening the overall investigation of the outbreak. Each state conducted case–control studies and identified alfalfa sprouts as a food item eaten by the cases in the seven days before the interview (the matched odds ratios were 27 in Michigan and 25 in Virginia, with 95% confidence intervals outside 1 in both outbreaks). In 29 instances out of 31 where persons had reported eating alfalfa sprouts, investigators were able to trace the alfalfa sprouts to the facilities that had sprouted the sprouts.

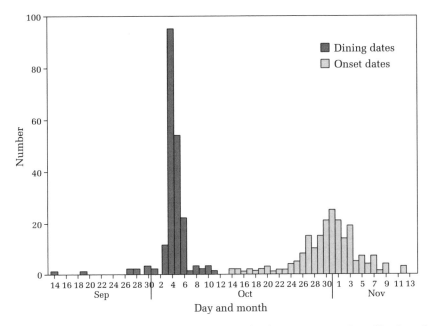

Figure 6-1. Number of hepatitis A cases by date of eating at restaurant A, and by date of illness onset: Monaca, Pennsylvania, 2003. $N = 206$; excludes one case-patient whose illness onset date was not available. Dining dates for three persons who ate at restaurant A on October 15 ($n = 1$) and October 17 ($n = 2$) are not shown. Source: Centers for Disease Control and Prevention (2003).

The tracebacks in Michigan led to one facility in Michigan with a possible second, and the tracebacks in Virginia led to one facility in Virginia. Both facilities used the same seed lot, and this seed lot was found to be a blend of five lots from four Idaho farms harvested between 1984 and 1996. The seed lot had totaled 17,000 lbs, and the 6,000 lbs still existing at the time of investigation were removed from distribution. Investigations at the farms identified several possible sources of contamination, including neighboring feedlots, water, and deer from a wildlife refuge, but the precise source of contamination was not conclusively determined. This outbreak is striking because of the long time period between growth of the seeds and consumption (1984–1997) and the widespread geographic distribution of the product.

Case Study 3: An Outbreak of Outbreaks—Parasitic Contamination of Raspberries

The two outbreaks described below were among 55 distinct events or outbreaks occurring between May 3 and June 14, 1996, and resulting in 725 cases of infection with *Cyclospora cayetanensis*, a coccidian parasite (Herwaldt et al.

1997, 1999; Caceres et al. 1998; Fleming et al. 1998). In May 1996, 101 guests attended a wedding reception in Boston, Massachusetts. Following the wedding reception, several attendees had diarrheal illness, and two were diagnosed with cyclosporiasis. The city health department initiated an outbreak investigation, beginning with a guest list of the wedding attendees. Thus, the investigators had already concluded that the illness had resulted from the wedding; in this type of outbreak, attendees often know each other, and the hosts are generally aware of illnesses among their guests. Had the attendees not suggested the wedding as a common source, the investigation would have taken a different course. Investigators calculated attack rates for each food item served at the wedding, based on guests' responses to a questionnaire. Because the outbreak took the traditional form (church supper scenario), the investigation followed the traditional methods of basing the exposure questionnaire on the foods served at the wedding reception, reconstructing the cohort of individuals who attended the wedding, and calculating attack rates for each food item (exposure). Table 6-1 summarizes the foods served, the attack rates for each food item, and the relative risk of illness for people who ate the food compared to people who did not eat the food. The relative risk was highest for people who ate the desert, berries and cream, compared to people who did not eat the desert (2.2; 95% confidence interval, 1.20–3.73).

On May 23, 1996, 64 people attended a woman's golf tournament luncheon at a country club in Charleston, South Carolina. Thirty-eight people became ill. Again, the outbreak followed the church supper scenario: attendees knew each other, spoke with each other, and quickly suspected that they had become ill by eating something at the luncheon. The South Carolina Department of Health and Environmental Control investigated the outbreak, identified *Cyclospora* oocysts in the patients stool samples, and conducted a retrospective cohort study to calculate attack rates for the foods served at the luncheon. The relative risk for was highest for eating raspberries (5.9; 95% confidence interval, 2.2–13.2).

Another 740 cases were identified, but not associated with any outbreak, bringing the total to 1,465 cases were reported in 20 states, the District of Columbia, and two provinces. Data were available for 41 events, and in 27 of these analyses, raspberries were associated with illness at statistically significant levels ($p < 0.05$). This outbreak of outbreaks triggered an investigation of its own, yielding a separate report in the *New England Journal of Medicine*. At the time this investigation was published, the authors hypothesized that "simultaneous and persistent contamination on multiple farms is the most likely explanation for the outbreak" (Herwaldt et al. 1997, p. 1554). They had not identified the source of *Cyclospora* and could not determine whether the oocysts came from humans or animals or whether they were unsporulated (on workers' hands) or had already sporulated (e.g., in the soil or water). The CDC

TABLE 6-1.   Attack rates and relative risk associated with exposures to various foods and beverages served at the wedding

Item	Exposed ill/total (%)	Unexposed ill/total (%)	Relative risk (95% confidence interval)
Ham	11/25 (44)	26/37 (70)	0.6 (0.4–1.0)
Turkey	19/34 (56)	16/26 (62)	0.9 (0.6–1.4)
Roast beef	16/22 (73)	20/89 (51)	1.4 (1.0–2.1)
Potato salad	16/19 (84)	20/42 (48)	1.8 (1.2–2.6)
Carrot and raisin salad	12/21 (57)	24/39 (62)	0.9 (0.6–1.5)
Pasta salad	10/29 (69)	17/34 (50)	1.4 (0.9–2.1)
Raspberries	33/37 (89)	4/24 (17)	5.4 (2.2–13.2)
Strawberries	34/49 (69)	1/13 (31)	2.3 (1.0–5.2)
Tea	17/31 (55)	21/33 (64)	0.9 (0.6–1.3)
Open bar	11/14 (79)	27/50 (54)	1.5 (1.0–2.1)

had not identified definitive reservoirs in animals, chickens, or birds. No oocysts were found in samples of water and raspberries tested on the farms.

The following year (1997), multistate, multicluster outbreaks of cyclosporiasis were again linked to Guatemalan raspberries (Herwaldt et al. 1999). Seven hundred and sixty-two cases were reported in 41 distinct outbreaks, and additional 250 cases, not associated with an outbreak, were reported separately. Although measures were put in place after the 1996 outbreaks to improve water quality, it is possible that the measures "were not fully implemented by some farms, were ineffective, or did not address the true source of contamination" (Herwaldt et al. 1999, p. 218). Tracebacks suggested that eight Guatemalan exporters had shipped the raspberries (figure 6-2). A number of farms in Guatemala provided raspberries to these exporters, and shipments combined raspberries from more than one farm, but the traceback could not clearly identify the farms where contamination must have taken place. On May 28, 1997, shipment of Guatemalan raspberries was suspended; no outbreaks of raspberry-associated cyclosporiasis were reported in the three months following the suspension of shipments (figure 6-3). In the spring of 1998, the FDA did not permit importation of fresh raspberries from Guatemala.

Case Study 4: An Outbreak Associated with Two Concurrent Bacterial Pathogens

A nursing home with a population of 580 residents reported an outbreak of diarrheal illness (Layton et al. 1997). One hundred and nineteen residents became ill, and 93 symptomatic patients submitted specimens. The laboratory results showed that 24 were positive for *Salmonella* Heidelberg, 14 were

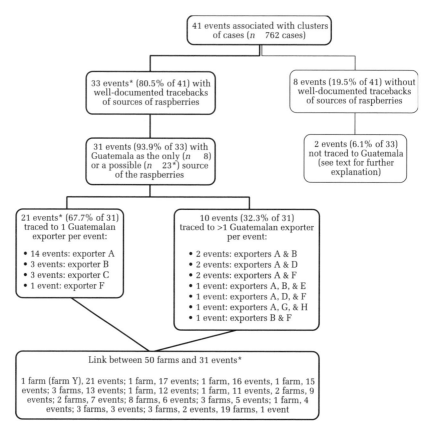

Figure 6-2. Tracebacks of sources of raspberries served at events associated with clusters of cases of cyclosporiasis in North America in 1997. *Includes three events (one traced to Guatemalan exporter A and two traced to Guatemalan exporter B) for which there might have been additional branches of the tracebacks without well-documented data; only well-documented data are included here. A farm was considered linked to an event if it contributed to a shipment of raspberries that could have been used at that event. Source: Herwaldt et al. (1999), used with permission of *Annals of Internal Medicine*.

positive for *Campylobacter jejuni*, and 25 were positive for both. The nursing home presents a unique set of challenges: six different dietary plans were available (regular, diabetic, low-salt, low-fat, soft, and pureed), and 125 food handlers were employed by the nursing home. Investigators used two case definitions: a broad definition including diarrhea and fever, and a definition for culture-positive cases only. The culture-confirmed cases also included asymptomatic residents with positive cultures, and included patients positive for one of six serotypes of *C. jejuni*, for *Salmonella* Heidelberg, or for both.

Arguments could be made in favor of broad or specific case definitions. A broad definition might be based on the hypothesis that a systematic error in-

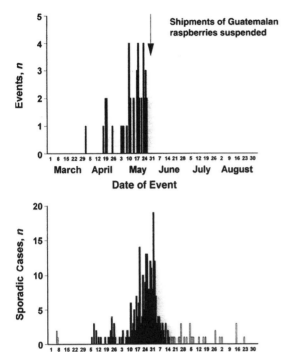

Figure 6-3. Dates of 41 events associated with clusters of cases of cyclosporiasis ($n = 762$ cases) in the United States and Canada in April and May 1997. For multiday events, the date of the first day of the event is shown. The last shipment of Guatemalan raspberries in the spring of 1997 was on May 28. Source: Herwaldt et al. (1999), used with permission of the *Annals of Internal Medicine*.

troduced multiple pathogens at one time, while the narrower definitions (dividing patients into subgroups) might be based on the hypothesis that two or more separate errors introduced pathogens within the same time period.

The epidemic curve seemed to suggest a point source; onset of cases clustered around two days, July 2 and 3. The investigators conducted a case–control study using the definition of culture-confirmed cases for their case group and drawing controls from the resident population. The analysis stratified the cases into three groups, culture positive for *C. jejuni* alone, *Salmonella* Heidelberg alone, or both. This stratification allowed the analysis to consider exposures associated with the subgroups or with the entire group. Five pureed meat and poultry items were most strongly associated with positive culture, but the analysis could not discriminate between the five items and could not detect associations with the specific pathogens. Investigators discovered that a food-handling error had occurred several days before: cooked chicken livers were processed in a meat grinder and placed in a bowl that contained juices from the raw liver. The following day, the refrigerator broke and the chopped chicken liver reached a temperature of 50°F. The case–control analysis did not distinguish chopped chicken liver from the four other foods associated with illness. It is possible that the other pureed products were contaminated through use of the same blenders or other equipment, and that individuals eating one pureed item also ate other pureed items and all ended up associated with illness. Perhaps multiple pathogens were introduced by various batches of chicken livers combined in one bowl.

As with many other outbreaks, the outbreak subsided without definitive confirmation of the food vehicle and food-handling errors but with rather strong pieces of supporting evidence. The statistical evidence derived from the analysis of the case–control study was less conclusive than results of other epidemiologic studies used to guide public health decision actions; however, the public health interventions in this outbreak were generic training in hand washing for the nursing home staff, monitoring staff for symptoms, and limiting group activities for symptomatic patients. The outbreak investigation paralleled the interventions rather than preceding them, and the interventions did not follow directly from the findings of the epidemiologic investigation.

Case Study 5: Intentional Contamination with a Bacterial Agent—*Salmonella* Contamination of a Salad Bar

Our one known example of intentional bacterial contamination causing a foodborne outbreak occurred in 1984 and was only reported in 1997 (Torok et al. 1997). This event preceded the heightened concerns about bioterrorism that followed the anthrax exposures and illnesses in 2001. Since the anthrax contamination, greater attention has been turned to the entire range of potential bioterrorism acts. An outbreak of *Salmonella* Typhimurium was observed in September and October 1984 in Oregon, and 751 persons with *Salmonella* gastroenteritis were identified. Most cases were associated with 10 restaurants, and eating from the salad bar was the major risk factor for illness. No particular food item, supplier, or distributor was common to all affected restaurants. A separate, criminal investigation found that members of a religious commune had contaminated the salad bars with bacteria grown in laboratories at the commune. The strain of *Salmonella* that infected people who ate at the salad bar was identical to that found in the commune's laboratory. The scientific investigation does not necessarily have the tools or authority to discover a criminal cause of contamination; however, the criminal investigation would rely on scientific evidence to some degree (e.g., information about bacterial strain, and elimination of other explanations). Thus, any outbreak investigation may ultimately be recognized as a criminal or terrorist activity, at which point the authority and investigation transfer to law enforcement authorities. Public health officers involved in food safety may be in a position to encounter and recognize criminal contamination or bioterrorism, but the ultimate responsibility for such investigations will move out of the food safety arena to the law enforcement arena. This is a rather new role for public health officials, and brings a new set of issues, but is in many ways outside the science of outbreak investigation.

Case Study 6: Intentional Contamination with a Chemical Agent

Intentional contamination is not limited to bacteria. On December 21, 1998, a county in California received reports of eight persons with nausea, vomiting, and dizziness within two hours of eating at a local restaurant (Buchholz et al. 2002). A second cluster of 11 cases was reported on January 2, 1999. After ruling out bacterial or viral illness, the case–control analysis found illness to be associated with increasing levels of salt. Odds ratios for increasing levels of salt exposure increased from 1.9 to 3.0 and 4.0 compared to the lowest level of salt exposure, providing evidence supporting a dose–response relationship, one of the criteria in establishing causality. A battery of laboratory tests were conducted on food and water samples, and a specimen of vomitus tested positive for methomyl, a toxic carbamate pesticide. The authors noted, "We relied initially on screening tests that did not focus on pesticides. It was difficult and time consuming to find a laboratory willing and able to do more specific tests for pesticides, including methomyl. Ultimately, it was not until 4 months into the investigation that we identified the responsible toxic agent" (Buchholz et al. 2002, p. 609). Methomyl was then found in the salt supply used by the restaurant. Methomyl is a restricted-use pesticide, and a registration with the county office is required before purchase. The county registry identified a registered user of methomyl who lived at the same apartment complex as cook A, and another user who was a relative of cook B. The pesticide company hired by the restaurant did not use methomyl in its biweekly treatments. The epidemiologic investigation was reported in the *Journal of the American Medical Association* (Bucholz et al. 2002), at which time a criminal investigation was ongoing. The scientific investigation established methomyl as the cause of illness but did not explain how and why it entered the restaurant salt supply; that remained for the police department.

Conclusions

While a percentage of outbreaks follow the classic pattern of a church supper or picnic, there are endless permutations of the events leading to a food-borne outbreak. Contamination (accidental or intentional) or failure to eliminate pathogens anywhere along the farm-to-table continuum may lead to food-borne outbreaks. Errors on the farm or in early stages of the farm-to-table continuum may result in a wider diffusion of cases over time and geography, while errors closer to the point of consumption generally are more limited in their occurrence within a shorter period of time or smaller geographic area. This general pattern can be complicated by variations; for example, a person visiting an area may eat at a local restaurant and then fly across the country to his or her home state and report the case in a completely different jurisdiction.

Food-borne outbreaks tend to die down because the contaminated food becomes consumed, or because the vehicle and pathogen are quickly recognized. In such cases, public health officials have a range of options from recall of food implicated in the outbreak to closing plants and restaurants. The authority to remove contaminated foods from the marketplace or to close manufacturing and food service establishments resides with local, state, and federal regulators (as discussed in chapter 13). Evidence gathered in an epidemiologic outbreak investigation may thus be used to justify legal actions such as recalls and closings, and epidemiologic evidence thus becomes a subject for contention in the legal area, especially when recalls or closings are contested. Epidemiologic concepts of causality then encounter legal principles of evidence creating one of the greatest challenges in food safety; the scientific and legal perspectives may not always be the same, yet they need to mesh if consumers are to be protected from eating contaminated foods.

Finally, the true cause of some outbreaks may remain unidentified for a variety of reasons. After the outbreak subsides and the contaminated food is disposed of, most public health workers have already moved on to the next outbreak or public health emergency. There is little time to follow up on unanswered questions or to confirm the leading hypotheses. There is little time to write up many outbreak investigations, and not all outbreaks generate enough interest to warrant published reports. As a consequence, some outbreaks do not get reported beyond the state level, and many outbreaks are not summarized in scientific documents in either a public database or the peer-reviewed literature. The outbreak investigation is not subject to criticism or analysis by peers; similarly, the methods, hypotheses, and conclusions are not questioned by peers. Reports that are published are available for scrutiny by scientific peers, policy makers, and the public, but we do not know how the published reports reflect the overall universe of published and unpublished investigations (this issue is discussed in chapter 7, when considering aggregation of data for policy making). As mentioned throughout this chapter, most food-borne outbreaks take place in a crisis atmosphere under intense time pressure. As a consequence, attention shifts rapidly from week to week as outbreaks recede or new ones are recognized. The skills and approaches of the acute outbreak investigation are quite different than those required for long-term analysis of aggregate data; in this situation, the epidemiologic approach more closely resembles that used in chronic epidemiology.

References

Associated Press. (2002, July 13). "Hospital flooded with food poisoning cases after church supper." *Boston Globe.*

Breuer, T., D. H. Benkel, et al. (2001). "A multistate outbreak of *Escherichia coli* O157:H7 infections linked to alfalfa sprouts grown from contaminated seeds." *Emerg Infect Dis* 7(6): 977–982.

Buchholz, U., J. Mermin, et al. (2002). "An outbreak of food-borne illness associated with methomyl-contaminated salt." *JAMA* 288(5): 604–610.

Caceres, V. M., R. T. Ball, et al. (1998). "A foodborne outbreak of cyclosporiasis caused by imported raspberries." *J Fam Pract* 47(3): 231–234.

Centers for Disease Control and Prevention. (2003). "Hepatitis A outbreak associated with green onions at a restaurant—Monaca, Pennsylvania, 2003." *MMWR Morb Mortal Wkly Rep* 52(47): 1155–1157.

Fleming, C. A., D. Caron, et al. (1998). "A foodborne outbreak of *Cyclospora cayetanensis* at a wedding: clinical features and risk factors for illness." *Arch Intern Med* 158(10): 1121–1125.

Herwaldt, B. L., M.-L. Ackers, et al. (1997). "An outbreak in 1996 of cyclosporiasis associated with imported raspberries." *N Engl J Med* 336: 1548–1556.

Herwaldt, B. L., M. J. Beach, et al. (1999). "The return of *Cyclospora* in 1997: another outbreak of cyclosporiasis in North America associated with imported raspberries." *Ann Int Med* 130(3): 210–220.

International Association of Milk, Food and Environmental Sanitarians, Inc. (1999). *Procedures to Investigate Foodborne Illness.* Des Moines, IA: Author.

Lasky, T., and P. D. Stolley (1994). "Selection of cases and controls." *Epidemiol Rev* 16(1): 6–17.

Layton, M. C., S. G. Calliste, et al. (1997). "A mixed foodborne outbreak with *Salmonella* Heidelberg and *Campylobacter jejuni* in a nursing home." *Infect Control Hosp Epidemiol* 18(2): 115–121.

Olsen, S. J., G. R. Hansen, et al. (2001). "An outbreak of *Campylobacter jejuni* infections associated with food handler contamination: the use of pulsed-field gel electrophoresis." *J Infect Dis* 183(1): 164–167.

Sails, A. D., B. Swaminathan, et al. (2003). "Utility of multilocus sequence typing as an epidemiological tool for investigation of outbreaks of gastroenteritis caused by *Campylobacter jejuni*." *J Clin Microbiol* 41(10): 4733–4739.

Torok, T. J., R. V. Tauxe, et al. (1997). "A large community outbreak of salmonellosis caused by intentional contamination of restaurant salad bars." *JAMA* 278(5): 389–395.

7

EPIDEMIOLOGIC STUDY DESIGNS

Tamar Lasky

Beyond the immediate concerns surrounding a food-borne outbreak, public health officials may wish to take actions to reduce the overall occurrence of food-borne outbreaks. This raises questions regarding the most efficient use of resources so that regulations have the greatest impact on reducing the risk of a food-borne outbreak. From farm to table, opportunities arise for contamination, multiplication of pathogens, or introduction of chemicals and additives. Neglect of proper processing and handling steps can result in missed opportunities to destroy pathogens present in the food and to minimize chemical contamination.

Measures to reduce the risk of food-borne illness take place at all points in the farm-to-table continuum, and it is of interest to identify points at which measures should be strengthened or added, and points where an intervention is redundant, ineffective, and/or too costly relative to its impact. These questions face policy makers and public health officials. Proponents of interventions such as raising *Salmonella*-free flocks of chickens (as is done in Sweden), inspecting each pig brought to slaughter to screen out *Trichina* (as is done in parts of Europe), irradiation of meat, restaurant inspection, and other measures attempt to predict the impact of their proposed intervention on rates of food-borne illness as part of the analysis necessary to convince policy makers to adapt their proposals (complete risk assessment and economic analysis consider other factors as well, as described in chapters 9 and 12). People disagree on the best course of action, and many stakeholders—growers, manufacturers, consumers, and others—object to the costs (financial and otherwise) involved in a specific intervention.

In order to assess the impact of an intervention on overall rates of food-borne illness, it is necessary to demonstrate a causal relationship between the proposed intervention and cases of food-borne illness and to estimate the number of cases attributable to the cause. Thus, policy makers and the public would ideally like to know how many cases of illness will be prevented by a specific measure. Epidemiologic studies can provide data about the strength of association between a risk factor and disease and, in some cases, the proportion of cases that would be reduced if an exposure is eliminated (attributable risk or attributable fraction).

Chapter 4 discussed the application of a multicausal model to questions of food-borne illness. The analogy to other multicausal diseases can be made. For example, multiple factors contribute to the occurrence of heart disease and mortality from heart disease, and multiple interventions contributed to the downturn in cardiovascular mortality that was observed in the late 1970s and early 1980s. Attribution of the downturn was possible only after substantial epidemiologic work had been done to describe the relationships between smoking, blood pressure, diet, cholesterol, improved coronary care, and other factors, and cardiovascular disease and mortality. In comparison, the epidemiology of food-borne illness has barely begun to attempt to attribute illness to specific interventions, causes, factors, or food products, and the databases and knowledge required to do so are barely in place.

The decades of work on complex, multicausal diseases such as cancer and heart disease have led to the development of research designs and statistical approaches that can be applied to the study of food-borne illness. The methods that may be most readily applied to food safety at the aggregate level are ecologic studies, meta-analyses, and case–control studies. Ecologic studies (correlations and comparisons) have been used to assess the impact of *Salmonella* testing of meats and poultry and overall occurrence of *Salmonella* infections in humans. Information from multiple outbreaks has been compiled to generalize about relative contributions of different foods and the occurrence of food-borne illness. Case–control studies have been used to assess the relative contributions of different foods and behaviors to overall occurrence of infections with a given pathogen.

Ecologic Correlations

Attempts to quantify levels of microbial pathogens in animal carcasses began in the mid-1990s and centered around *Salmonella* testing at slaughter houses.

The government agency that inspects meat, the U.S. Department of Agriculture (USDA) Food Safety and Inspection Service, collects sample carcasses, swabs the carcasses, and conducts microbiologic analyses to detect the presence or absence of *Salmonella* and its subspecies. The test results are recorded in a newly developed database (MARCIS), which, although developed for enforcement rather than exposure measurement requirements, suggests to some scientists the feasibility of correlating levels of *Salmonella* found in animal carcasses with annual occurrence of human illnesses caused by *Salmonella*. If bacterial levels in animal products are a primary cause of food-borne illness, then one expects the two figures to be strongly correlated. This assumes that each measure—the measure of exposure, or pathogen levels in animal products, and the measure of disease, or reported, culture-confirmed cases of salmonellosis—is accurately measured. It also assumes that pathogen levels are relatively unchanged between production and consumption—that cooking, heating, storage, and handling are not significantly modifying the pathogen levels originating with the animal. It also assumes that the reported, culture-confirmed cases of salmonellosis include relatively few cases of non-food-borne salmonellosis (e.g., cases acquired through water, pets, or person-to-person contact).

Epidemiologists are well aware that ecologic correlations are the weakest type of evidence regarding causality; nonetheless, ecologic studies have generated interesting hypotheses and suggested important routes of inquiry. When attempting to correlate, for example, a measure of exposure (pathogen levels) with a measure of disease (reported cases), it is necessary to have confidence in both measures and in the assumptions made in hypothesizing a correlation. Even then, ecologic correlations do not directly link the exposure to the persons with disease. For example, national measures do not demonstrate that the persons with culture-confirmed cases of salmonellosis actually consumed any animal products whatsoever, or that their salmonellosis was acquired through consumption of any particular food product.

The recent political debate over *Salmonella* testing of animal products has dimensions outside the scope of epidemiology—whether the USDA has the authority to conduct such tests, whether the tests are markers or indicators for other pathogens, whether test results provide cause for government intervention, and what levels of positive (bacteria present) results should lead to government intervention. The existence of the database, although not intended as a measure of exposure, has nonetheless led politicians to inquire whether *Salmonella* test results are increasing or decreasing, and these results, in turn, are being interpreted as causally related to findings in trends in cases of illness. Epidemiologists who enter this debate may be able to help define the limits of the data, as well as point out directions for refinement of the data.

If some epidemiologists might be reluctant to link pathogen levels in animal products to disease levels in humans, others have suggested that the information can be used further to link serotypes of *Salmonella* observed in animal products to cases occurring in humans and to attribute cases of food-borne illness to specific animal products. Hald and Wegener (1999) present Danish data on *Salmonella* serotype distributions in humans, pork, beef, broiler chickens, and layer flocks and then present their estimates of the proportions of *Salmonella* cases arising from pork, beef, eggs, broilers, other poultry, unknown, and acquired outside of Denmark, but they do not provide details of their statistical methods. They then estimate the proportions of cases of salmonellosis in Denmark in 1998 associated with specific commodities in Denmark, or with travel outside of Denmark (figure 7-1). While they provide estimates of proportions of infections originating in different sources, they do not provide information on the production, processing, or food-handling steps that led to exposure and infection (whether products were undercooked or improperly refrigerated, whether handling of animal products resulted in contamination of vegetables or fruits, etc.), so the attribution has limited application in prevention and control of food-borne illness. Further, they may be able to attribute infections to food groups in Denmark, a relatively small and closed system, but it is not clear that a similar approach is feasible in the United States.

As the pathogen becomes defined more specifically, it may become more feasible to link the animal reservoir to the human cases. Nauerby et al. (2000),

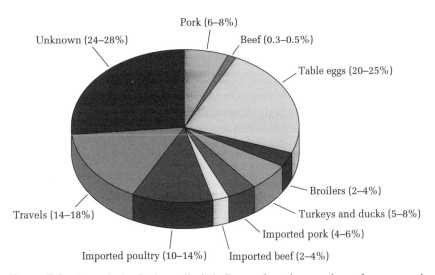

Figure 7-1. An analysis of salmonellosis in Denmark, and proportions of cases associated with different commodities in Denmark, 2000. Source: Ministry of Family and Human Affairs, Danish Institute for Food and Veterinary Research, Copenhagen, Denmark (2000). Annual report on zoonoses in Denmark 2000. Used with permission, Danish Zoonoses Center.

again in Denmark, isolated 10 strains of *Salmonella enterica* serovar Enteritidis phage type 11 (PT11) and six strains of PT9a from hedgehogs during
1994–1998, and identified five patients infected with PT11 and two with PT9a.
By further analyzing the isolates using pulsed-field gel electrophoresis, they
concluded that the strains from the hedgehogs and the humans belong to the
same clonal lineage. Carried to this level of detail, variation in serovar, strain,
phage type, and genetic sequence might serve as a tool to untangle the various sources of food-borne illness, but the approach is at an initial stage of
development. Another Danish example traced an outbreak of a strain of *Salmonella enterica* serotype Typhimurium known as definitive phage type 104
(DT104) that is resistant to five drugs (ampicillin, chloramphenicol, strepto-
mycin, sulfonamides, and tetracycline) to one particular herd of swine (Molbak
et al. 1999). Again, the specificity with which the investigator could characterize the pathogen, and its relative rareness, allowed linkage between animal source
and human illness. Whether these methods can be reliably applied to aggregate
data from large countries such as the United States has not been fully demonstrated, and the factors affecting application and validity of the methods have
not been laid out. These methods are mentioned here as subjects for future study
and investigation, but they are not ready for off-the-shelf use, nor are we yet
able to rely on microbiologic data to correlate pathogen levels in animals with
proportions of human illnesses caused by a given pathogen.

Information Gained from Outbreaks

If one wishes to know the overall most frequent causes of outbreaks, one might
tote up causes across outbreaks. One could look at the pathogens, the food
item, and the steps (or missteps) associated with each outbreak. Summarizing
across outbreaks is an intuitively appealing approach to understanding the
causes and consequences of food-borne outbreaks. Several groups have made
attempts to summarize information from multiple outbreaks and have relied
on databases maintained by various government agencies.

Since 1973, the Centers for Disease Control and Prevention (CDC) has
maintained a database describing reported food-borne outbreaks (the Food-
borne Disease Outbreak Surveillance System) and has summarized data peri-
odically in the *CDC Surveillance Summary* (Centers for Disease Control and
Prevention 2000). Defining food-borne outbreaks as "two or more cases of a
similar illness resulting from the ingestion of a common food," the CDC documented 2,751 such outbreaks between 1993 and 1997. The database provides
information for each outbreak on the number of cases and deaths, state reporting the outbreak, month of occurrence, foods implicated, and place where food
was eaten. It also contains information on outbreaks caused by chemical con-

tamination, such as ciguatoxin, heavy metals, and monosodium glutamate. Data for 1993–1997 show, for example, that 23.8% of reported outbreaks were associated with a bacterial pathogen, 5.4% with a chemical contaminant, 0.7% with a parasitic agent, and 2.0% with a viral agent, but 68.1% were of unknown etiology. The data are also summarized by place where food was eaten. In 1997, out of 481 outbreaks where the place where the food was eaten was known, 113 were associated with a private residence, 216 with a delicatessen, cafeteria, or restaurant, 17 at a school, 6 at a picnic, 10 at a church, 4 at a camp, and 115 at some other place. The Center for Science in the Public Interest maintains a database of outbreaks that appears to be a subset of the CDC database, supplemented with information derived from other sources, and categorizes outbreaks by the food item and the agency responsible for regulating the food item (DeWaal et al. 2001). They include only outbreaks with an identifiable etiology or vehicle.

In England and Wales, outbreaks are summarized in the National Surveillance Database for General Outbreaks of Infectious Intestinal Disease. Lopman et al. (2003a) used the data to group *Norovirus* outbreaks by site, comparing outbreaks in residential homes and hospitals institutions to outbreaks in other settings, and found differences in the seasonal distribution of outbreaks (figures 7-2 and 7-3). In another analysis, Lopman et al. (2003b) summarized and compared viral outbreaks in 10 different European surveillance systems. They demonstrated variation in surveillance definitions, populations under surveillance, and completeness of descriptive and analytic epidemiologic and diag-

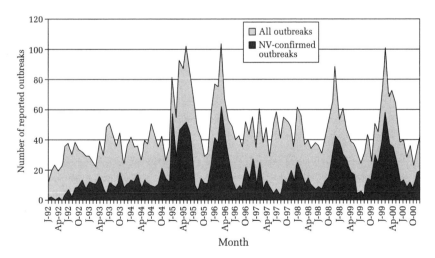

Figure 7-2. Seasonality of all outbreaks and confirmed *Norovirus* outbreaks, England and Wales, 1992–2000. Source: Lopman et al. (2003a).

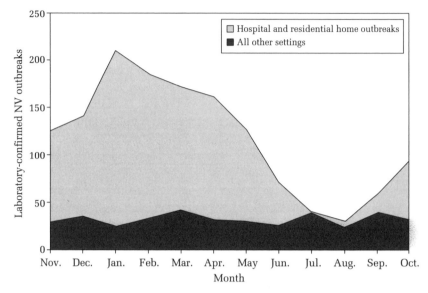

Figure 7-3. Seasonality of *Norovirus* outbreaks in residential homes and hospitals compared to all other settings, England and Wales, 1992–2000. Source: Lopman et al. (2003a).

nostic information. When methods vary to this degree, it may not be possible to summarize findings across systems.

Summarization of such data across outbreak reports is analogous to meta-analysis of observational studies or of clinical trials (see further discussion of meta-analysis in chapter 8). However, the highly rigorous methodology of meta-analysis has not yet been fully applied to the task of summarizing across outbreaks. Two methodologic issues are of critical concern: biases leading to reporting (or nonreporting) of outbreaks, and quality of information reported. Although surveillance systems such as the CDC's Foodborne Disease Outbreak Surveillance System should ideally ensure a nonbiased ascertainment of outbreaks, state reporting of outbreaks to CDC appears to be highly variable. State and local health departments vary in their response to outbreak reports and in the resources available for outbreak investigations, and this variation may contribute to differences in reporting. For example, between 1993 and 1997, Washington State reported 5–30 times more outbreaks of foodborne illness per capita than did Oregon, and 12 times more than California (Centers for Disease Control and Prevention 2000).

The biases introduced by reporting differences have not been fully explored or documented. One could hypothesize that the worst outbreaks receive the most attention and are thus reported, but it is also possible that severe outbreaks occur in states with poor resources and low reporting rates. Comparison of outbreak surveillance in England and Wales to published reports indicates a bias favoring publication of novel outbreaks (O'Brien et al. 2002). Further work is needed to examine these and other hypotheses. The CDC has recently implemented a web-based reporting system (Electronic Foodborne Outbreak Reporting System [EFORS]), but it is not clear whether this has resulted in more complete and consistent reporting of outbreaks. In March 2002, the CDC presented data showing the number of outbreaks reported by year, before and after EFORS was implemented. From 1997 to 1998 (EFORS initiated in 1998), outbreaks reported increased from 806 to 1,314 (figure 7-4). The following two years, reports remained high at 1,344 and 1,380, but by 2001 reports decreased to 1,026, higher than before EFORS was implemented but lower than the first three years of implementation. From these data, one cannot tell whether reporting has increased, or whether the number of reports reflects an actual change in the number of outbreaks. It is also not possible to determine how many outbreaks have not been reported and what factors are associated with reporting of outbreaks. In order to generalize from multiple outbreaks, one requires a sample of outbreaks that reflects the universe of all outbreaks or, at least, the ability to identify the universe of outbreaks. At present, this is not possible. This is a critical issue in attempting to use aggregate data about outbreaks to shape public policy. Exploration of the factors associated with outbreak reporting would be helpful to better understand the contribution and limitations of the available summaries of reported outbreaks.

Even when outbreaks are reported to the CDC or similar authority in another country, they are not always accompanied by a publicly available text document similar to a journal publication. Scientists interested in conducting a systematic literature review or a meta-analysis may not have access to data and

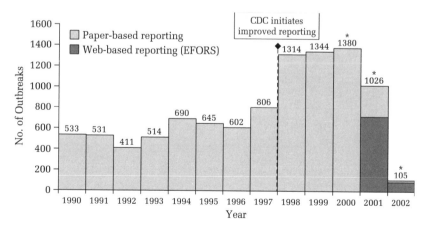

Figure 7-4. Number of outbreaks reported to the CDC through the Foodborne Disease Outbreak Surveillance System as of March 15, 2002. In June 2001, the CDC completed development of EFORS. Source: Centers for Disease Control and Prevention (2003).

information needed to assess the methodology of the outbreak investigation and the quality of the evidence. Some outbreaks are reported in peer-reviewed journals, but it is not clear what percentage of outbreaks is published. While the CDC database contains mention of 5–600 outbreaks a year, a search of Medline shows fewer than 50 food-borne outbreaks published in a given year. Again, the factors leading to publication of food-borne outbreaks are unknown. In contrast to other fields of epidemiology, one would not expect publication bias associated with negative findings (no effect) because an outbreak, by definition, describes an effect. Instead, other factors may play a bigger role in determining whether an outbreak is written up, submitted, accepted, and published in the peer-reviewed literature. Some outbreaks may not be written up and published if they appear routine and thus not considered as a scientific contribution. Other factors, such as the time demands of the investigator or an institution's aversion to negative publicity, may also discourage publication. To date, no one has conducted a meta-analysis or systematic literature review of the published studies or attempted to understand the factors leading to publication of reports of food-borne outbreaks. Before using aggregated outbreak reports to estimate the role of various factors contributing to food-borne illness, it is essential to describe the target universe of food-borne outbreaks and the selective factors that result in an outbreak entering a database of food-borne outbreaks, from recognition to reporting, to publishing. This is an example where the food safety field will be able to draw on the methodology developed by epidemiologists addressing other public health problems.

A further problem in summaries of outbreaks is a tendency for analysis to shift between the units of study, beginning perhaps with the outbreak as the unit of study, and shifting to individual cases as the unit of study. The total number of cases is a function of outbreak size, which is partially a function of the point at which errors or contamination take place. An error in handling food in the home will generally result in fewer cases than an error in handling food at a catering establishment or restaurant; the size of the outbreak, or the number of cases, is a function of the number of people who consume the food but does not necessarily mean that one food holds more risk than another. When analyzing outbreaks, it is probably best to maintain the outbreak as the unit of analyses and develop statistical methods for incorporating individual case information.

Case–Control Studies

Population-Based Case–Control Studies

Another form of aggregate study is the case–control study, comparing unrelated cases of food-borne illness (called "sporadic" in some studies) to controls, people without the food-borne illness. Investigators increasingly use population-based case–control studies to identify general factors associated with the probability of becoming infected. In the population-based case–control study, individuals may have acquired their infections through various pathways, vehicles, and routes of transmission. This is in contrast to the use of case–control studies within an outbreak investigation, when one assumes a common source, pathway, and exposure. Examples of population-based case–control studies include studies of salmonellosis in Spanish children, *E. coli* O157:H7 in the United States and in Belgium, campylobacteriosis in England, cholera in Ecuador, listeriosis in the United States, and toxoplasmosis in pregnant women in Europe and Scandinavia (Schuchat et al. 1992; Ikram et al. 1994; Weber et al. 1994; Kapperud et al. 1996; Willocks et al. 1996; Eberhart-Phillips et al. 1997; Mead et al. 1997; Blasco et al. 1998; Delarocque-Astagneau et al. 1998; Slutsker et al. 1998; Baril et al. 1999; Pierard et al. 1999; Cook et al. 2000; Rodrigues et al. 2001; Hunter et al. 2004).

These studies compare cases to controls with respect to eating habits, recalled dietary intake, and other factors such as owning pets, visiting farms, or traveling abroad, and estimate the risk associated with each factor by calculating an Odds Ratio (Box 7-1). This is a fascinating example of a concept

---

BOX 7-1

The case–control study design was developed in the 1950s to address the difficulties in studying diseases with relatively low incidence rates and long time periods between exposure to a causal factor and the occurrence of disease. Case–control studies ask how people with the disease are different from people without the disease.

The researcher identifies people with the disease (case) and a group of comparison people without the disease (controls) and collects information about each person's risk factors and exposures. For each risk factor or exposure studied, data are entered into a two-by-two table, and an odds ratio and its 95% confidence interval are calculated.

	Number of persons with disease (cases)	Number of persons without the disease (controls)
Number of persons with risk factor or exposure	a	b
Number of persons without risk factor or exposure	c	d

Odds ratio = $a \times d / b \times c$

taken from chronic disease epidemiology and applied to infectious diseases. Ironically, the approach of studying multiple risk factors in chronic disease epidemiology was originally viewed as inconsistent with the concepts of causality that had been developed in infectious disease epidemiology. The adaptation of the population-based case–control study to the study of heterogeneous cases of food-borne illness may require more thought and attention to methodologic issues. Sophisticated statistical analysis is required to assess the interrelationship among variables such as education and social class, potential risk factors such as food-handling practices or eating in restaurants, and accompanying risk factors for non-food-borne acquisition of "commonly food-borne" pathogens (e.g., water supply or pet ownership). In particular, accurate estimates of effect (odds ratios) and of attributable risk associated with specific food groups or handling practices may require further work.

Case–Control Studies to Identify the Causes of Food-Borne Illness: The Example of Toxoplasmosis

Toxoplasma gondii is parasitic protozoan that can infect all warm-blooded animals and birds. *T. gondii* has three infective stages in its life cycle: (1) sporozoites released from oocysts in feline feces; (2) tachyzoites, the forms that infect animal cells and multiply rapidly; and (3) bradyzoites, forms that are encysted in animal tissue and organisms. The oocysts excreted by cats can persist in water and in soil; thus, there are several potential routes of exposure: through ingestion of contaminated water, exposure to cat feces (e.g., when changing the kitty litter), and handling and consumption of animal tissue (meat and poultry) infected with *T. gondii* (Smith 1993). The disease is not transmitted from human to human, except through maternal transmission to the fetus.

Infection with *T. gondii* is quite common: the Third National Health and Nutrition Examination Survey (1988–1994) showed that 22.5% (95% confidence interval, 21.1–23.9) of the population were seropositive for immunoglobin G antibodies to *T. gondii* (Jones et al. 2001). Infants and the immunosuppressed may experience severe consequences as a result of *Toxoplasma* infection. The most recent study of congenital toxoplasmosis comes from the New England Newborn Screening Program between 1986 and 1992, 635,000 infants underwent serologic testing, and 52 were infected, an infection rate of approximately 1/10,000 live births (Guerina et al. 1994). Follow-up of 48 infected infants found that 19 (48%) had signs of disease, including abnormal cerebrospinal fluid examinations, hydrocephalus, and retinal lesions. Because of concerns about permanent damage to the infant, including blindness, many public health efforts regarding toxoplasmosis are directed toward pregnant women. Another group greatly affected by toxoplasmosis is immunosuppressed persons. Toxoplasmosis is an AIDS-defining opportunistic infection and is frequently the immediate cause of death in HIV-infected persons, in whom it causes severe illness, toxoplasmic encephalitis, and death.

Tables 7-1 and 7-2 summarize the characteristics and results from four case–control studies testing hypotheses regarding risk factors for toxoplasmosis. Three of the studies focus on risk factors in European pregnant women (France, Norway, and a six-country multicenter study), and one study focuses on risk factors in farm workers in Illinois (Kapperud et al. 1996; Baril et al. 1999; Weigel et al. 1999; Cook et al. 2000). The sample sizes for the case group ranged from 54 to 252, and in three of the studies, multiple controls were collected for each case. Each study began with fairly lengthy lists of potential risk factors or exposure variables (18–44 variables) and similar groups of variables referring to eating habits (particularly eating raw foods), hygiene, contact with animals (with emphasis on cats), gardening, and travel. The number of variables related to each group varied: the study by Weigel et al. (1999) asked about handling of raw meat but did not ask about eating raw meat. In contrast, the study by Cook et al. (2000) asked 15 questions about meats eaten, their frequency, and state of rawness.

The case–control studies confirmed that infection with toxoplasmosis is associated with consumption of raw meats or vegetables, contact with an infected cat or its litter, contact with soil, and poor hygiene (infrequent washing of knives), and these associations are consistent with our understanding of the organism *T. gondii* (biologic plausibility). Thus, two criteria for causality are present: a fairly strong, statistically significant association is observed in epidemiologic studies, and the association is biologically plausible. The studies collected data on different foods (and food groupings) and found different foods to be strongly associated with infection. In one study, undercooked beef was the meat most

TABLE 7-1   Characteristics of case–control studies of risk factors for toxoplasmosis

Reference	Population	Number of cases	Number of controls	Number of risk factors tested
Baril et al. (1999)	Pregnant women, France	80	80	29
Weigel et al. (1999)	Farm workers, Illinois (USA)	54	120	18
Cook et al. (2000)	Pregnant women, six European countries	252	708	30
Kapperud et al. (1996)	Pregnant women, Norway	63	128	44

TABLE 7-2   Results of case–control studies of risk factors for toxoplasmosis

Reference	Risk factors*	Odds Ratios
Baril et al. (1999)	Undercooked beef	5.5
	Pet cat	4.5
	Raw vegetables eaten outside home	3.1
Weigel et al. (1999)	Cat inside pig facilities	0.32
	Handle pig feed	0.36
	Number of seropositive cats on farm	1.1
	Gardening	2.18
	Pigs raised on pasture	3.88
	Patient's sex	3.97
Cook et al. (2000)	Raw/undercooked beef	1.73
	Raw/undercooked lamb	3.13
	Other meat	4.12
	Taste meat cooking	1.52
	Contact with soil	1.81
	Travel outside Europe/US or Canada	2.33
Kapperud et al. (1996)	Eating raw or undercooked minced meat	4.1
	Eating unwashed raw vegetables or fruits	2.4
	Eating raw or undercooked mutton	11.4
	Eating raw or undercooked pork	3.4
	Cleaning the cat litter box	5.5
	Washing the kitchen knives infrequently	7.3

*Variables whose odds ratios had 95% confidence intervals that did not include 1.

strongly associated with infection; in a second study, other meat (not lamb or beef) was most strongly associated with infection, and in a third study, raw or undercooked mutton was the meat most strongly associated with infection. Where the studies found similar meats as risk factors, the odds ratios differed widely, as in the example of raw or undercooked lamb or mutton, for which the odds ratio was 3.13 in one study and 11.4 in another study.

The question for policy makers is whether the estimates of the association observed in case–control studies can be used to quantify the relative contribution of each of these different factors (attributable risk). The attributable risk concept has been most applied in chronic disease epidemiology, where repeated, multiple exposures accumulate and affect the occurrence of cancer or heart disease. Thus, one can attempt to calculate the proportion of cancers attributable to air pollution versus the proportion of cancers attributable to pesticide exposures. However, problems in interpreting case–control data have been well described. Estimates of odds ratios are greatly affected by the underlying distributions of potential exposures, the other exposures studied and entered in the statistical models, the choice of controls, and correlations within the group of variables. Food habits, in particular, are highly correlated with numerous factors such as culture, education, socioeconomic status, and lifestyle, which in turn are correlated with water supply, hygiene, housing, occupation, health care of family, immigration status, and so on.

Attributable Risk

Attributable risk is the difference in the risk of disease in a population if an exposure or risk factor is eliminated, and the attributable fraction is the proportion of cases that would not occur if the exposure or risk factor was reduced or eliminated. This is most readily estimated when an exposure falls into a few discrete groupings, and is strongly associated with disease (e.g., smoking). Unfortunately, diets and eating habits are extremely complex and varied and are difficult to measure and categorize (as described in chapter 5), and food-borne illness can be categorized along many parameters. Food-borne outbreaks have been categorized by pathogen, vehicle (food carrying the pathogen), site of consumption (home, restaurant, institution), and type of error leading to outbreak. Cases not linked to an outbreak are generally categorized by pathogen only, with little investigation into the factors suspected of causing the case.

There has been some interest in identifying the proportion of illness associated with a specific food or food group. For each food of interest, points along the farm-to-table continuum can be identified for potential intervention. However, interventions at most points may reduce illness caused by foods other than (or in addition to) the one of interest, resulting in an overall decrease in illness but no change in the proportion associated with a particular food. Interventions are often promoted by agencies or organizations responsible for a particular product; it is reasonable, then, that they wish to demonstrate that the proportion (and absolute numbers) of illnesses related to their product has gone down as a result of their efforts. The many steps from farm to table, the complex interrelationships among steps along the way, and the many foods that have been associated with food-borne illness make this a daunting task. While population-based case–control studies have been undertaken to identify risk factors for food-borne illness, they have not been able to estimate precisely the contribution of different foods to the overall occurrence of food-borne illness. The task of attributing cases to specific foods has been more difficult than some expected (Batz et al. 2005).

Case–Control Studies with Restaurants as the Unit of Study

The case–control study design developed by epidemiologists over the past 50 years compares individuals with illness (cases) to individuals without the illness under study (controls). A novel twist on this method has been the use of studies that compare restaurants with unfavorable outcomes (food-borne outbreaks) to restaurants without the unfavorable outcomes. In such studies, the restaurant is the unit of study, and while it may seem logical to apply the case–control method to the study of restaurants, the methodologic issues involved in such an application have not been explored.

In a study in Seattle and King County in Washington State, 28 restaurants with a food-borne outbreak in the study period were compared to 56 restaurants with no history of food-borne outbreaks in the same study period, with respect to inspection records prior to the time period of interest (Irwin et al. 1989). The authors found that poor inspection scores were predictive of a food-borne outbreak and, in particular, that violations of proper temperature controls of potentially hazardous foods were associated with occurrence of a food-borne outbreak. A similar study in Miami and Dade County in Florida compared inspection reports of 51 restaurants with outbreaks in 1995 to 76 restaurants without outbreaks and found no association between overall inspection outcome or mean number of critical violations (Cruz et al.2001). They found that one violation, evidence of vermin (odds ratio = 3.3; 95% confidence interval, 1.1–13.1), was associated with occurrence of outbreaks. Many factors can be hypothesized to explain the difference in findings; for example, the inspection processes may not be the same in each county, the definition of outbreak might not be identical, or different variables may have been included in each analysis. Of even greater importance is that of fully applying epidemiologic thinking to the problem of comparing restaurants. How would confounding be defined, and how would one control for confounding in this context? Would size of the restaurant be a confounding variable? (Do larger restaurants have a higher risk of outbreak occurrence?) What is the best metric for restaurant size—number of customers, number of meals, number of square feet? What about the ratio of physical space to number of meals? If size plays a role in risk of outbreak occurrence, how would one adjust for size in statistical analysis? Perhaps it is necessary to weight the findings for each restaurant by the size of the restaurant to adjust for the effect of size; perhaps other adjustments are needed.

It is exciting that public health researchers are making new uses of epidemiologic concepts and applying epidemiologic designs to new contexts; at the same time, great caution must be taken in interpreting the results of these new applications. This presents a challenge to epidemiologists, that of meeting the unique requirements in studying food safety questions. It may also require patience from the food safety community and the public, as methodologic challenges are explored and solutions developed.

References

Baril, L., T. Ancelle, et al. (1999). "Risk factors for *Toxoplasma* infection in pregnancy: a case-control study in France." *Scand J Infect Dis* 31(3): 305–309.

Batz, M. B., M. P. Doyle, et al. (2005). "Attributing illness to food." *Emerg Infect Dis* 11(7): 993–999.

Blasco, J. B. B., J. M. G. Cano, et al. (1998). "Factors associated with sporadic cases of salmonellosis in 1- to 7-year old children: study of cases and controls." *Gac Sanit* 12(3): 118–125.

Centers for Disease Control and Prevention. (2000). "Surveillance for foodborne-disease outbreaks—United States, 1993–1997." *CDC Surveillance Summaries* 49(SS-1).

Centers for Disease Control and Prevention. (2003). Foodborne-disease outbreaks reported to CDC January 1, 1990 through March 15, 2002. Atlanta, GA, Author.

Cook, A. J., R. E. Gilbert, et al. (2000). "Sources of *Toxoplasma* infection in pregnant women: European multicentre case-control study. European Research Network on Congenital Toxoplasmosis." *BMJ* 321(7254): 142–147.

Cruz, M.A., Katz, D.J., Suarez, J.A. (2001) "An Assessment of the Ability of Routine Restaurant Inspections to Predict Food-Borne Outbreaks in Miami-Dade County, Florida, *Am J Public Health*, 91(5) pp 821–823

Delarocque-Astagneau, E., J. C. Desenclos, et al. (1998). "Risk factors for the occurrence of sporadic *Salmonella* enterica serotype enteritidis infections in children in France: a national case-control study." *Epidemiol Infect* 121(3): 561–567.

DeWaal, C. S., K. Barlow, et al. (2001). Outbreak alert! Washington, DC, Center for Science in the Public Interest.

Eberhart-Phillips, J., N. Walker, et al. (1997). "Campylobacteriosis in New Zealand: results of a case-control study." *J Epidemiol Community Health* 51(6): 686–691.

Guerina, N. G., H. W. Hsu, et al. (1994). "Neonatal serologic screening and early treatment for congenital Toxoplasma gondii infection. The New England Regional Toxoplasma Working Group." *N Engl J Med* 330(26): 1858–1863.

Hald, T., and H. C. Wegener. (1999). "Quantitative assessment of the sources of human salmonellosis attributable to pork." Paper presented at the Third International Symposium on the Epidemiology and Control of *Salmonella* in Pork, Washington, DC, August.

Hunter, P. R., S. Hughes, et al. (2004). "Sporadic cryptosporidiosis case-control study with genotyping." *Emerg Infect Dis* 10(7): 1241–1249.

Ikram, R., S. Chambers, et al. (1994). "A case control study to determine risk factors for campylobacter infection in Christchurch in the summer of 1992–3." *N Z Med J* 107(988): 430–432.

Irwin, K., Ballard, J. et al. (1989) "Results of routine restaurant inspections can predict outbreaks of foodborne illness: the Seattle-King County experience." *Am J Public Health* 79(5): 1678–1679.

Jones, J. L., D. Kruszon-Moran, et al. (2001). "*Toxoplasma gondii* infection in the United States: seroprevalence and risk factors." *Am J Epidemiol* 154(4): 357–365.

Kapperud, G., P. A. Jenum, et al. (1996). "Risk factors for *Toxoplasma gondii* infection in pregnancy. Results of a prospective case-control study in Norway." *Am J Epidemiol* 144(4): 405–412.

Lopman, B. A., G. K. Adak, et al. (2003a). "Two epidemiologic patterns of norovirus outbreaks: surveillance in England and Wales, 1992–2000." *Emerg Infect Dis* 9(1): 71–77.

Lopman, B. A., M. H. Reacher, et al. (2003b). "Viral gastroenteritis outbreaks in Europe, 1995–2000." *Emerg Infect Dis* 9(1): 90–96.

Mead, P. S., L. Finelli, et al. (1997). "Risk factors for sporadic infection with *Escherichia coli* O157:H7." *Arch Intern Med* 157(2): 204–208.

Ministry of Family and Human Affairs, Danish Institute for Food and Veterinary Research, Copenhagen, Denmark (2000). Annual report on zoonoses in Denmark 2000. Copenhagen: Danish Zoonosis Center.

Molbak, K., D. L. Baggesen, et al. (1999). "An outbreak of multidrug-resistant, quinolone-resistant *Salmonella enterica* serotype Typhimurium DT104." *N Engl J Med* 341(19): 1420–1425.

Nauerby, B., K. Pedersen, et al. (2000). "Comparison of Danish isolates of *Salmonella enterica* serovar Enteritidis PT9a and PT11 from hedgehogs (*Erinaceus europaeus*) and humans by plasmid profiling and pulsed-field gel electrophoresis." *J Clin Microbiol* 38(10): 3631–3635.

O'Brien, S. J., I. A. Gillespie, et al. (2002). "Examining publication bias in foodborne outbreak investigations: implications for food safety policy." Paper presented at the Conference on Emerging Infectious Diseases, Atlanta, GA, Centers for Disease Control and Prevention.March 24–27 2002.

Pierard, D., N. Crowcroft, et al. (1999). "A case-control study of sporadic infection with O157 and non-O157 verocytotoxin-producing *Escherichia coli*." *Epidemiol Infect* 122(3): 359–365.

Rodrigues, L. C., J. M. Cowden, et al. (2001). "The study of infectious intestinal disease in England: risk factors for cases of infectious intestinal disease with *Campylobacter jejuni* infection." *Epidemiol Infect* 127(2): 185–193.

Schuchat, A., K. A. Deaver, et al. (1992). "Role of foods in sporadic listeriosis. I. Case-control study of dietary risk factors. The Listeria Study Group." *JAMA* 267(15): 2041–2045.

Slutsker, L., A. A. Ries, et al. (1998). "A nationwide case-control study of *Escherichia coli* O157:H7 infection in the United States." *J Infect Dis* 177(4): 962–966.

Smith, J. L. (1993). "*Toxoplasma gondii* in meats—a matter of concern?" *Dairy Food Environ Sanit* 12(6): 341–345.

Weber, J. T., E. D. Mintz, et al. (1994). "Epidemic cholera in Ecuador: multidrug-resistance and transmission by water and seafood." *Epidemiol Infect* 112: 1–11.

Weigel, R. M., J. B. Dubey, et al. (1999). "Risk Factors for Infection with *Toxoplasma gondii* for residents and workers on Swine Farms in Illinois." *Am J Trop Med Hygiene* 60(5): 793–798.

Willocks, L. J., D. Morgan, et al. (1996). "*Salmonella* virchow PT 26 infection in England and Wales: a case control study investigating an increase in cases during 1994." *Epidemiol Infect* 117(1): 35–41.

8

DATA QUALITY

Tamar Lasky

Data quality is an issue for epidemiologists at all times, but the rapid growth and use of food safety risk assessment create new challenges in evaluating data quality. As discussed in chapter 9, a risk assessment may require multiple data sources to estimate a single step in a risk analysis, and an even greater number of data sources for the entire risk assessment. The demand for data is coupled with an increasing availability of data sets, all with varying quality. Epidemiologic principles can be applied to identify, evaluate, and combine data as inputs to a food safety risk assessment. Indeed, epidemiology in the areas of exposure measurement and disease measurement has developed extensive methods for estimating data points. In addition, epidemiology in the specialized area of meta-analysis has also developed methods for combining estimates of effects across more than one study. These principles are well known to epidemiologists reading this text; for food scientists and risk assessors new to epidemiology, some key concepts are summarized in this chapter.

The purpose of this chapter is to provide principles and resources for risk assessors in food safety to identify information to be used in risk assessment, develop procedures for decisions regarding inclusion or exclusion of information from risk assessments, and combine estimates from more than one study to produce measures to use in risk assessment models. These processes are similar to those used in meta-analysis; however, in many risk assessments, the stringent conditions of meta-analysis cannot be met. The methodology developed to conduct meta-analyses can be adapted and applied to the needs of risk assessment, with the eventual goal of raising the quality of information used. The methodology developed for meta-analysis can even be used by risk assessors to address problems when the data are of poor quality or do not meet the criteria for meta-analysis; a systematic literature review can be conducted by following many of the principles developed for meta-analysis and identifying areas where data are inadequate. A systematic review may be defined as "a review that has been prepared using a systematic approach to minimizing biases and random errors which is documented in a materials and methods section. A systematic review may, or may not, include a meta-analysis: a statistical analysis of the results from independent studies, which generally aim to produce a single estimate" (Egger et al. 1997, 2001, p. 5; Egger and Smith 1997).

Data Quality Guidelines

Risk assessors and policy makers struggle formally with data quality issues in the peer-reviewed literature, as well as in the courts and in the political process. This does not discount the importance of data quality in outbreak investigations, surveillance, case–control studies, and other food safety activities, but use of epidemiologic data in risk assessment and policy brings in a wider group of stakeholders and intense scrutiny of the data. The subject of data quality has received increasing attention from risk assessors, policy makers, regulators, and the government, with all parties attempting to provide guidelines and set standards for data quality.

Discussions about data quality have taken place in a number of settings, and epidemiologists have contributed greatly to the general discussions, but it is not clear that there is general agreement of data quality principles or a widespread understanding about evaluation of data quality. The World Health Organization (WHO) guidelines for use of epidemiological data in health hazard characterization and in health impact assessment present processes and approaches to assess epidemiological information for environmental risk assessment (World Health Organization Working Group 2000). They address studies assessing causal relationships between an exposure and effect and, in addition, address studies that supply estimates of population exposures and behaviors, either as point estimates or as interval estimates. The guidelines stress the importance of adopting a systematic and explicit approach to the assessment of epidemiologic evidence for health risk assessment, including development of a protocol for the review, comprehensive identification of all relevant studies (and documentation of methods used to identify all relevant studies), systematic assessment of the validity of epidemiological studies, and the use of meta-analysis to provide overviews of the evidence from multiple studies (World Health Organization Working Group 2000).

A nonprofit organization, Federal Focus, Inc., based in Washington, DC, has held a series of discussions regarding the use of epidemiologic data in science policy, and in risk assessment in particular. Their first publication, *The Role of Epidemiology in Regulatory Risk Assessment*, considered issues involved in evaluating individual studies as well as a body of literature and is directed toward environmental or chemical risk assessment (Graham 1995). It is most applicable to studies describing an association, as would be required in hazard identification of a chemical exposure. A follow-up document, designated the "London Principles," resulted from a three-day conference in London and emphasizes epidemiologic evidence, epidemiologic studies, and assessment of causality for environmental or chemical risk assessment (Federal Focus, Inc. 1996). The principles echo basic epidemiologic principles but are not easily implemented. They employ subjective qualifiers, such as "sufficient detail," "biologically sound," "properly quantitated," "clearly defined," and "properly measured," which are not objectively defined. An underlying assumption appears to be that a fully trained epidemiologist will be part of the risk assessment process:

> The principles are intended for use primarily by government risk assessors who are preparing a complete risk assessment for probable use in a significant regulatory decision; however, the risk assessors should include, or be assisted by, expert epidemiologists, and ideally, also by experts from other relevant disciplines such as medicine, toxicology, and biostatistics. (Federal Focus, Inc. 1996, p. 9)

A further problem in implementing these guidelines is that they were heavily critiqued (but not resolved) in follow-up documents (Federal Focus, Inc. 1999). An expert panel was assembled to review the London Principles by attempting to apply them to a specific body of literature, studies of possible association between induced abortion and breast cancer. The exercise led to suggestions for changes to the principles and indications of areas that need revision. Unfortunately, this effort has not been followed by any conclusive solution incorporating the criticism. The principles are thus not readily implemented as usable guidelines. The discussion provides a list of questions for supervising risk assessors and risk management officials to ask the epidemiologists and other risk assessment team members; the questions assume an interdisciplinary team that includes epidemiologists (Federal Focus, Inc. 1999).

The Office of Information and Regulatory Affairs in the U.S. government's Office of Management and Budget (OMB) implements the Data Quality Act (2002), enacted to ensure that all information disseminated by the federal government is reliable. Whether data quality can or cannot be regulated depends on many factors, including widely agreed upon and understood standards for data quality. Food safety scientists may need to acquire a deeper understanding of data quality issues and draw epidemiologist more deeply into their work. General guidelines, principles, and discussions are not a substitute for a well-grounded understanding of sampling, data collection, variable definition, and other features of epidemiologic data. They provide an excellent resource for risk assessors in microbial risk assessment, but they are not easily applied to food safety risk assessment, for the following reasons: (1) the greatest attention has been devoted to chemical/environmental risk assessment issues; (2) in many cases, the discussions assume that a doctoral-level epidemiologist will be a key member of the risk assessment team and principles for evaluating epidemiologic data are often not translated into a format that can be applied by scientists with less epidemiologic training; (3) the discussions focus on studies of causality (hazard identification and measures of effect) but do not provide guidance on studies that are used to provide point estimates of an exposure or disease; and (4) the discussions focus on one or more stages in the process of formulating a question, identifying the data sources, and evaluating and combining the data but do not attempt to provide guidelines for the entire process.

Much can be gained from studying the work that has been done in chemical and environmental risk assessment, and much of what has been done is readily applicable to microbial risk assessment. However, a greater effort is needed to identify areas that are applicable and issues that are unique to microbial risk assessment. Food safety risk assessments require a variety of data and information inputs, and it would be valuable to develop guidelines that apply to information gathering and synthesis throughout a risk assessment, whether this involves "animal data," "survey data," "epidemiologic data," or other types. Finally, it is useful to address the entire process in one document; data searches, data evaluation and quality, and data synthesis are interrelated and strongly tied to the type of question being addressed.

Identifying Data for Use in Risk Assessment

Defining the Question, Measurement, or Data Point Needed

It may be self-evident that the first step is to define the question before searching for reports and studies (table 8-1), but relatively little has been written about this step. Light and Pillemer (1984) devote several pages to the issue of formulating a precise question in their chapter on organizing a reviewing strategy, but their examples are drawn from the clinical arena of treatment evaluations and clinical guidelines. In a food safety risk assessment, a conceptual model of the factors affecting food safety is expressed as a mathematical model, and information is collected and combined for each step in the model. A comprehensive food safety microbial risk assessment might model processes from farm to table in order to inform food safety policy. For example, a risk assessment of *E. coli* O157:H7 in ground beef might include steps designated by the broad terms—grinding, storage (retail), transportation, storage (home), and cooking—and risk assessors might proceed to collect information regarding each of these steps. Before beginning library and other searches, it might be useful to specify details for each of the steps and to articulate the precise scientific question that underlies the inclusion of the step in the model. As shown below, taking time to delineate specific questions can provide focus and direction for the information gathering process.

In a food safety risk assessment model, the step labeled "cooking" may be specified (figure 8-1): How does cooking modify the number of live pathogens present in a specified portion of food? How frequently do the different effects occur? Cooking can result in a range of effects on pathogen levels, totally eliminating live bacterial pathogens at high temperatures or multiplying and increasing pathogen levels at low temperatures. The initial conceptual questions thus require information about the number of possible cooking behaviors (which itself may be defined by several variables such as time, temperature, method, or amount of food), the frequency with which these behaviors occur, and some measure of the effect of each behavior on live microbial pathogen levels. To address these questions, we would need to conduct at least three separate search and evaluation processes to identify appropriate information:

1. How has cooking of the food product been categorized in the scientific literature (and for what purposes)? For example, cooking can be categorized by method (frying, boiling, roasting, etc.), length of time (in minutes or hours), temperature reached, and type of utensils (grill, microwave, toaster). If there is more than one categorization scheme cited in the literature, the data may not be comparable, and the risk assessor will need to decide what scheme is most appropriate for the risk assessment. In

TABLE 8-1   Steps for identifying and synthesizing information from multiple data sources.

Step 1. Define question, measurement, or data point needed.
Step 2. Identify primary sources of data with information about question, measurement, or data point.
Step 3. Evaluate data sources for inclusion or exclusion, and document decision-making process.
Step 4. Combine information across data sources through formal meta-analysis or other approach.

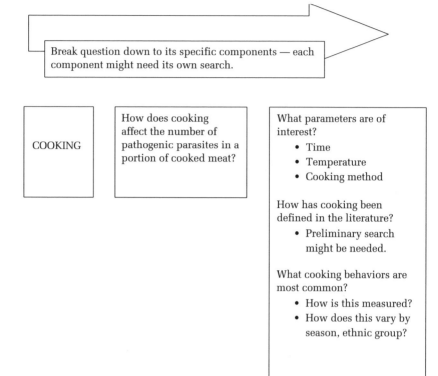

Figure 8-1. Before searching or combining data, define the question in as much detail as possible. A risk assessment model might have a step labeled "cooking," and this can be broken down into several questions.

addition, the number of categories produced by different schemes will affect the precision of the data and its usefulness in risk assessment.

2. How frequent are the different behaviors relative to each other, relative to total consumption of the food product, and (perhaps) relative to total food consumption behaviors? After identifying categorization schemes, it will be feasible to combine data from different studies only if they use equivalent categorization schemes. Data from a study categorizing cooking by time and temperature will not be easily combined with data from studies categorizing cooking by method (frying, boiling, etc.).

3. How do the cooking behaviors affect live microbial pathogen levels in food (in quantitative terms)? This might require data from laboratory studies testing the effects of different methods, times, and temperatures on pathogen levels in the specified food.

Multiplying the frequencies in item 2 by the effects in item 3 will produce an overall estimate of the effect of cooking on pathogen levels in the foods in question, but the validity of the categorization scheme in item 1 and the number of categories will affect the precision and accuracy of estimates of the effect. What began as one question can be broken down into three (or more) different questions, each requiring a data identification, evaluation, and synthesis process.

Search Strategies

The search for information needs to emphasize comprehensiveness and systematic criteria for identifying relevant sources. Complete comprehensiveness is rarely attained and not always required (figure 8-2). Many searches automatically exclude non-English-language sources, unpublished sources, and/or sources published before a given date. In many cases, these are reasonable exclusions; however, it is again important to articulate the exclusions, for accuracy in documentation and transparency and for evaluating the suitability of the exclusions. While it may be acceptable to exclude non-English-language sources for risk assessments for U.S. policy, it is probably not valid to exclude them in risk assessments for European or world policy. If one opens the criteria to allow non-English-language sources, some rationale needs to be offered for the languages included, and the criteria need to be applied in a systematic manner.

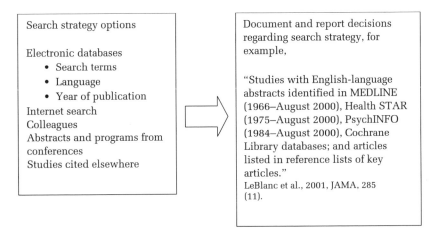

Figure 8-2. Search strategies can take various forms, but whatever decisions are made about materials to be searched or excluded, clear documentation is needed for each search undertaken for each of the component questions.

In conducting a search for information and data, decisions are made, implicitly or explicitly, regarding year of publication, published versus nonpublished references, choice of reference databases, and search terms. From habit or convenience, one may choose to search a given reference database, and by definition this will exclude references before a certain date and will exclude nonpublished references. Whether this is done out of habit, convenience, or deliberate decision making, it needs to be documented, applied consistently, and justified to some degree. It is reasonable to apply cutoffs by year of publication; however, the choice of the year may vary by specific scientific question. In some fields, 10 years is about as far back as one would go, but in other fields, especially where data are scarce, one might go back considerably further. As a current example, the scarcity of human anthrax cases in the United States prior to 2001 required public health officials to scour literature from the 1950s and 1960s, much further back in time than one generally goes when considering clinical data.

Unpublished Data

Decisions regarding unpublished data are especially controversial. Arguments in favor of using unpublished data state that data are more likely to be published if results differ from the null and that published data therefore are biased away from the null (Sutton et al. 2000). Publication bias is especially well studied regarding clinical trials. When performing a meta-analysis of clinical trials, it is therefore essential to identify unpublished studies. One may ask colleagues, scan conference proceedings and lists of dissertations, and contact funding organizations, government agencies, or industry to identify and obtain the results of unpublished clinical trials (Abramson and Abramson 2001). While clinical trial meta-analysts advocate the use of unpublished studies, environmental epidemiologists have raised questions about documentation and quality of unpublished data. The Committee on Environmental Epidemiology of the National Research Council, along with the Commission on Life Sciences, issued the report *Environmental Epidemiology: Use of the Gray Literature and Other Data in Environmental Epidemiology* in 1997. The committee concluded that most studies in the gray literature of environmental epidemiology (state health department reports, doctoral and master's theses, and reports produced by special interest groups) have serious limitations. The committee reviewed the use of "studies that are available to the public but not published in the indexed scientific and technical literature" with respect to environmental or chemical risk assessment. Their main conclusion regarding the gray literature was that "most studies and reports in the gray literature have serious limitations, such as lack of adequate exposure information, that seriously undermine their credibility and value. However, the gray literature may contain studies and reports that point to directions for further research or that contain the only information on a topic" (Committee on Environmental Epidemiology and Commission on Life Sciences 1997, pp. 174–175).

Given the strong arguments for and against the use of unpublished studies in meta-analysis and risk assessment, it appears necessary to identify and evaluate unpublished data and then decide whether to include them, and to describe the rationale for inclusion or exclusion from a risk assessment. In many cases, it will be necessary to conduct a search that includes unpublished sources; however, the results of such a search may not necessarily lead to inclusion of the unpublished sources in the risk assessment. Rather, the reviewer might document that unpublished sources were reviewed, specify the unpublished sources reviewed, and describe the justification for excluding the reviewed sources from the literature synthesis.

Documenting the Search Strategy

A comprehensive search may include more than one bibliographic database and may attempt several combinations of search terms. It is worthwhile to run a series of searches and combine the reference lists to eliminate duplicates. For example, one might search on various combinations of "infections," "*Salmonella* infections," "gastrointestinal infections," "food-borne illness," and so on, when looking for references regarding food-borne salmonellosis. Literature search skills and requirements vary by scientific discipline, but the process has grown increasingly sophisticated in the past decades. Excellent software options are available for managing this process and will also produce the necessary formatted bibliography. The time and skills involved in managing the search and obtaining, filing, and reviewing references may require planning for personnel dedicated to this process. Again, documentation of the search terms, strategies, and databases is essential.

After conducting a search, one obtains a list of references. This list can be thought of as a database itself, with n entries. After removing duplicate entries, the n of the database is the number of individual references collected according to the criteria discussed above. At this point in a search, the n may be several-fold (even 10-fold) larger than the number of documents that are finally used in the risk assessment, because one attempts to cast a wide net and pull in anything that is relevant. A preliminary review of the references can be done relying on the abstracts. Broad criteria can be used to exclude references that do not appear to be relevant. Again, consistency and documentation are key to a transparent and systematic approach. In summarizing the process, one should be able to describe the number of references that were excluded and the reasons for excluding them (e.g., "23 references were excluded because they were animal studies," or "12 references were excluded because they did not address bacterial pathogens"). The references that remain are then evaluated for data quality and inclusion in the risk assessment.

As stated in the preceding sections, data are excluded from risk assessments either explicitly, in articulated decisions, or implicitly, by assumptions governing the search process. A key principle is that exclusions and inclusions need to be documented and described. After conducting a search and implementing broad exclusions (e.g., based on publication dates or language), one assembles a group of studies containing original scientific data regarding the specific step in the model. These data will vary greatly in quality, and the question arises of how to decide which data to use in the risk assessment model. The question is particularly problematic in areas with relatively little research and where data may not be as high quality as desired. Whether a decision is made to include or exclude the data from a risk assessment, it is important to discuss the data quality, its limitations, and its possible effect on the model. This increases the transparency of the risk assessment process and leads to a clear identification of future data needs.

When information is abundant, the risk assessor can set up guidelines for inclusion following principles outlined in discussions of epidemiology and meta-analysis and exclude data that do not meet criteria for quality. The principles followed should be documented and cited, applied to each data source, and summarized somewhere in the risk assessment document (either in the document itself or in an appendix). A summary table or matrix is useful in describing the criteria as applied to each data source. Matrices can be simple or complex; in either case, they permit quantification and documentation of the characteristics of the articles reviewed, excluded, and included in the literature synthesis. When information is scarce, the risk assessor may not be able to implement criteria for quality. In this situation, the risk assessor needs to acknowledge and describe data quality limitations. Some risk assessors will prefer to include poor-quality data, while mentioning its limitations; others will prefer to exclude poor-quality data and model clearly stated assumptions. In either case, the decision needs to be discussed and documented.

Evaluating Data Quality

Much of the literature on meta-analysis and research synthesis applies to studies of causality or association. In many steps of a risk assessment model, estimates of mean levels or proportions and their confidence intervals are needed, without measures of effect. Microbial risk assessments draw on a variety of data sources at each step in the model, including data regarding industrial processes, laboratory microbiological data, animal data, survey data, infectious disease incidence rates, outbreak investigation reports, and dose–response data. The concepts discussed below are relevant to all data types but are particularly important in assessing data collected about human beings, data that most frequently come from observational studies where the researcher has much less control over study subjects compared with laboratory studies. Epidemiologists do not generally work with animal data; however, the principles below can be applied to animal data, and risk assessors, epidemiologists, veterinarians, and food safety professionals will need to work together to apply the principles to animal data. Decisions to include or exclude data from a risk assessment can be made in the context of the following concepts. Definitions from Last (1995) are provided as starting points for discussion. The definitions were developed to be applicable to a broad range of scientific fields. The concepts are basic, discussed in the biostatistics and statistics literature, and are applicable to all data (figure 8-3).

Generalizability, Representativeness

The more similar the study population is to the population targeted by the risk assessment, the more relevant the use of the study data.

Representativeness is defined by Last (1995) as follows: "The term *representative* as it is commonly used is undefined in the statistical or mathematical sense; it means simply that the sample resembles the population in some way" (p. 146). Data sources should provide information about the population that was studied or sampled. Animal populations can be described by biological species, age, sex, and so on, and human populations can be defined by time period of data collection, geographic unit, age groups, sex, race/ethnicity, mental status (as in studies of dementia or Alzheimer's dis-

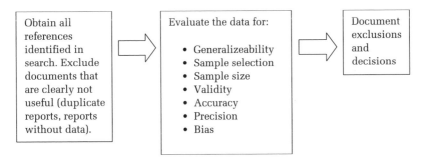

Figure 8-3. After conducting the search, a subgroup of documents are evaluated for data quality and requirements of the risk assessment. Again, decisions are made regarding exclusions and inclusions, and the decisions are documented.

ease), listed/unlisted telephone numbers, institutionalization, medical conditions, and many other characteristics. The risk assessor needs to judge whether the study population characteristics are similar to the population targeted by the risk assessment and, if not, whether the dissimilarity invalidates the value of the data source.

Sample Selection

Random-probability–based samples are preferable to self-selected or convenience samples.

A sample is "a selected subset of a population. A sample may be random or nonrandom and may be representative or nonrepresentative" (Last 1995, p. 150). Sampling strategies affect the ability to infer characteristics of the larger, underlying target population based on the study sample. Random samples are the ideal in most cases. Nonrandom samples may be highly selective and introduce a variety of biases. A data source should provide information about its sampling strategy and its effects on study findings.

Sample size

Estimates from large sample sizes are more precise than estimates from small sample sizes.

Sample size affects the precision of the estimate produced from the data. Small sample sizes produce imprecise estimates with wide confidence intervals. Large sample sizes produce estimates with narrower confidence intervals, decreasing uncertainty in the risk assessment.

Validity

Validated operational measures are preferable to unvalidated or questionable measures.

Concepts of validity can apply to individual measurements or to an entire study. Measurement validity is "an expression of the degree to which a measurement measures what it purports to measure" (Last 1995, p. 171). Study validity is "the degree to which the inference drawn from a study, especially generalizations extending beyond the study sample, is warranted when account is taken of the study methods, the representativeness of the study sample, and the nature of the populations from which it is drawn" (p. 171). Particularly when studying humans, we cannot measure exactly what we would like to measure.

For example, one may wish to measure the temperature meat is stored in the home refrigerator, but instead of taking actually temperature measurements of individual home refrigerators, one might ask respondents what temperature they keep their refrigerator at. This latter measure is valid only if it can be demonstrated that individuals are knowledgeable about their refrigerator temperatures and accurate in reporting the temperatures to an interviewer. In this example, a concept, "refrigerator temperature," is operationalized as a survey question. The validity of the survey question as an operational measure of the concept "refrigerator temperature" is unknown. If the operational measure is not valid, then the data collected will not be useful and can be quite misleading.

Accuracy

Accuracy in the data increases the predictive ability of the model.

Accuracy is "the degree to which a measurement or an estimate based on measurements represents the true value of the attribute that is being measured" (Last 1995, p. 3). The accuracy of a data measurement is affected by validity of the measurement tool and sources of bias but is also affected by the mechanics of data collection. Data recorded electronically can be subjected to automatic edit checks ensuring completeness and decreasing improbably values. Electronic methods also eliminate the need for data entry from the paper-and-pencil format, reducing transcription errors. In general, electronic data collection methods are less prone to error than are pencil-and-paper methods; however, errors in programming can introduce errors in electronic data collection, as well. Checks of data quality and accuracy can be conducted and measured quantitatively by resampling a subsample of the study. Measures of accuracy can be provided with documentation accompanying the data set.

Data regarding humans are often collected using some type of survey instrument, whether in an actual survey or as part of some other study design such as a cohort study, case–control study, or clinical trial. In each of these different designs, questionnaires and/or interviews in person, in writing, over the telephone, or self-administered can be conducted to gather baseline and follow-up information. Large public databases are also highly dependent on survey technology and vary greatly in sophistication. Survey design and administration are a highly researched areas with extensive literature addressing data accuracy. A risk assessor concerned about the accuracy of information in a survey database may wish to consult an expert in survey methodology when evaluating the data quality.

Precision

Increases in data precision lead to decreases in uncertainty and variability in the model.

Precision is "the quality of being sharply defined through exact detail. A faulty measurement may be expressed precisely but may not be accurate. Measurements should be both accurate and precise, but the two terms are not synonymous" (Last 1995, p. 128). Precision is affected by the intervals used to measure a variable, the study instrument, coding, data entry, and chemical and physical limits of detection/measurement. As an example, age in surveys is often defined in broad categories such as younger than 18, 18–64, and 65 or more years of age, but it can be defined more precisely in years, and even more precisely in months, weeks, and days, as when studying infants, and even hours and minutes, as when studying newborns.

Bias

Bias in data estimates used in a risk assessment decreases the predictive value of the risk assessment model.

As defined by Last (1995), bias is a "deviation of results or inferences from the truth, or processes leading to such deviation; any trend in the collection, analysis, interpretation, publication, or review of data that can lead to conclusions that are systematically different from the truth" (p. 15). An extensive epidemiologic literature describes different sources of bias, types of bias, effects of bias, and methods of correcting for bias. Sources of bias can be grouped as measurement errors, sample selection and study design, response/refusal, and data completeness. Measurement errors may be systematic over- or underestimates of true value because of bias in the measurement tool. Questionnaires are particularly prone to measurement errors if questions are worded in ways that suggest responses (i.e., "Do you ever drink too much?" vs. "How much do you drink?"). Sample selection and study design can systematically leave out or oversample a sector of the population. A historic example is the telephone survey in attempting to predict the outcome of the 1948 U.S. presidential election. By definition, it left out people who did not own telephones (people who also had lower incomes and were more likely to vote Democratic) and thus erred in its prediction of the outcome. Differential response and/or refusal rates can bias results; if response rates are low, the respondents may not be representative of the target population, and the same applies if refusal rates are high. Data completeness is somewhat related to the issue of response rates. With long survey instruments or telephone interviews, respondents tend to get bored or quit before completion; however, this can also vary with the quality of the form and of the interviewer and with the motivation for participation (compensation or other). If a specific sector of the target sample quits in mid-interview, or does not return for follow-up questions, a bias may be introduced.

Combining Data from More Than One Study: Meta-Analysis

The term "meta-analysis" can be used in both a broad and a narrow sense. In the broadest sense, meta-analysis refers to everything discussed in this chapter —defining a question, identifying data sources, setting criteria for inclusion and exclusion of data, and combining and contrasting information. In the more narrow sense, meta-analysis refers to the statistical issues involved in combining estimates from more than one study. If several sources of data are identified for use in a risk assessment, it may be necessary to combine the information from the multiple studies. Much of the methodology originally developed for statistical meta-analysis (documenting search strategies, developing objective criteria for inclusion, etc.) is applicable to systematic literature reviews and the broadest definitions of meta-analysis. The combining of estimates from more than one study raises specific statistical issues that are addressed briefly below (see figure 8-4). In such analyses, the ultimate goal is to calculate an overall effect or measure by combining the data, and this calculation would feed directly into a risk assessment.

An arithmetic average of study results does not account for the greater variance in small studies; thus, it is appropriate to use a weighted average giving large studies more influence than small studies. Two types of models are used in these calculations: the "fixed-effects" model and the "random-effects" model. The fixed-effects model assumes that variability between studies is exclusively due to random variation. The random-effects model assumes a different underlying effect for each study and accounts for this additional source of variation, leading to wider confidence intervals than for the fixed-effects model. Bayesian models are available for either of the above models and, again, may increase the width of the confidence interval. The individual results from multiple studies can be graphed and compared to the results achieved after meta-analysis (figure 8-5). The resulting estimate is more precise (has a smaller confidence interval) and reflects the findings of each of the studies included.

Assessment of the heterogeneity between study results can be challenging. On the one hand, as heterogeneity increases, it becomes less clear that study results can be combined. However, if no heterogeneity exists, it is hardly necessary to go through the exercise of meta-analysis. It becomes necessary to conduct statistical tests for heterogeneity across studies. Less heterogeneity permits the fixed-effects assumption, while greater heterogeneity may require

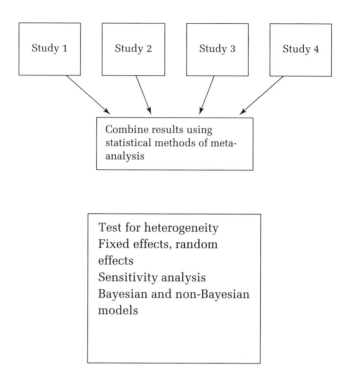

Figure 8-4. Some use the term "meta-analysis" to denote the statistical methods for combining results from more than one study.

the random-effects assumption. Furthermore, the heterogeneity needs to be examined for differences that may explain the heterogeneity of results.

The meta-analysis can be conducted under differing assumptions: (1) for both fixed- and random-effects models, (2) applying varying criteria regarding quality of studies, and (3) stratifying by sample size to assess publication bias—if publication bias is present, the largest sample sizes will produce the smallest effects. Conducting these different analyses allows one to assess the robustness of the findings to choice of statistical method and decisions regarding data quality.

Planning Meta-Analyses or Systematic Literature Reviews

Guidelines and recommendations for conducting meta-analysis and/or systematic literature reviews increasingly call for explicit development of a protocol guiding the conduct of the meta-analysis and/or systematic literature review, as well as documentation of methodology and transparent reporting (Stroup et al. 2000). Several authors have pointed out that detailed planning, searching, and documentation may consume more resources than previously allot-

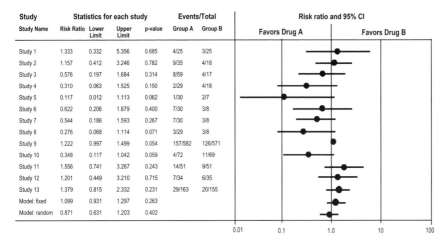

Figure 8-5. Meta-analysis: graph of individual study results, their 95% confidence intervals, and the combined measures of effect. The odds ratio and the 95% confidence intervals are plotted on a logarithmic scale so that 0.5 and 2.0 are equidistant from 1.0 (no effect), and confidence intervals are symmetrical around the point estimate. The results for each study are presented from top to bottom, and the combined effects are at the bottom. The size of the black squares marking the point estimate indicates the weight given to each study. Source: Metaworks, Inc., used with permission.

ted to literature searches. Egger et al. (1997) suggest that standardized forms be developed for recording information from the articles and that two independent abstractors extract the data to avoid errors. They also suggest a method of blinding abstractors to the names of the authors and their institutions, names of journals, and so forth, all of which require a substantial investment in time to conceal identifying information, photocopy and/or scan texts, and prepare standardized formats. Again, this requires planning and allocation of resources, time, and personnel.

Allen and Olkin (1999) provide estimates of the time involved in conducting meta-analysis, based on their firm's experience with 37 meta-analyses. They break the work into four categories and provide means and standard deviations of hours involved (table 8-2). The authors acknowledge the variability in different meta-analyses, as well as the increased efficiency with larger meta-analyses. They provide a formula for estimating hours based on the approximate number of citations gathered in a broad initial search.

A number of published guidelines provide formats for reporting meta-analysis and/or systematic literature reviews. The *Journal of the American Medical Association* format for reporting meta-analyses can be used in summarizing literature reviews and meta-analyses for risk assessment. In the *JAMA* structured abstract format (box 8-1), the question to be addressed

TABLE 8-2   Estimates of the number of hours of work at each stage of a meta-analysis.

Stage of work	Mean number of hours	Standard deviation
Preanalysis search, retrieval and database development —protocol development, searches, library retrieval, abstract management, study matrix construction, paper screening and blinding, data extraction and quality scoring, data entry, and data matrix construction	588	337
Statistical analysis	144	106
Report and manuscript writing	206	125
Other (administrative)—proposal development, project specific correspondence, project meetings and administration, project management and training	201	193

Source: Allen and Olkin (1999).

defines the objective for the systematic review and/or meta-analysis. This directly suggests a format for reporting and summarizing the information gathering process and conclusions in a risk assessment. One might write up a structured summary for each of the questions addressed at each step in the model. The process for evaluating data for inclusion in the risk assessment can then take place relative to the question being asked at each step in the risk assessment model.

The checklist presented by Stroup et al. (2000) may be one of the most useful to risk assessors, because it has been adapted for observational (nonclinical trials) studies (box 8-2). The authors present a checklist of items to address when reporting a meta-analysis of observational studies in epidemiology (not clinical trials). The authors include academic experts as well as government scientists, and by broadening the checklist to address nonclinical trials, they have increased its relevance to food safety risk assessment. The checklist can easily be adapted to improve the transparency of risk assessments. Following the checklist format, reports of data searches and synthesis can be included in text or appendices of risk assessments.

Epidemiologists working in food safety may be brought in because of their traditional experience in outbreak investigation, but skills in evaluating, aggregating, and combining data from different sources make the epidemiologist a key member of teams working on risk assessment and policy development. Methods of analysis have been developed that are applicable to the needs of food safety risk assessors and policy makers. Active collaboration between epidemiologists and food safety scientists is needed to adapt these methods to the particular challenges of the food safety arena.

BOX 8-1 *JAMA* Guidelines for Reporting Systematic Reviews or Meta-Analyses

Manuscripts reporting the results of meta-analyses should include an abstract of no more than 300 words using the following headings: Context, Objective, Data Sources, Study Selection, Data Extraction, Data Synthesis, and Conclusions. The text of the manuscript should also include a section describing the methods used for data sources, study selection, data extraction, and data synthesis. Each heading should be followed by a brief description:

Data Sources

Succinctly summarize data sources, including years searched. The search should include the most current information possible, ideally with the search being conducted within several months before the date of manuscript submission. Potential sources include computerized databases and published indexes, registries, abstract booklets, conference proceedings, references identified from bibliographies of pertinent articles and books, experts or research institutions active in the field, and companies or manufacturers of tests or agents being reviewed. If a bibliographic database is used, state the exact indexing terms used for article retrieval, including any constraints (e.g., English language or human subjects). If abstract space does not permit this level of detail, summarize sources in the abstract including databases and years searched, and place the remainder of the information in the Methods section.

Study Selection

Describe inclusion and exclusion criteria used to select studies for detailed review from among studies identified as relevant to the topic. Details of selection should include particular populations, interventions, outcomes, or methodological designs. The method used to apply these criteria should be specified (e.g., blinded review, consensus, multiple reviewers). State the proportion of initially identified studies that met selection criteria.

Data Extraction

Describe guidelines used for abstracting data and assessing data quality and validity (e.g., criteria for causal inference). The method by which the guidelines were applied should be stated (e.g., independent extraction by multiple observers).

Data Synthesis

State the main results of the review, whether qualitative or quantitative, and outline the methods used to obtain these results. Meta-analyses should state the major outcomes that were pooled and include odds ratios or effect sizes and, if possible, sensitivity analyses. Numerical results should be accompanied by confidence intervals, if applicable, and exact levels of statistical significance.

BOX 8-2 Table. A Proposed Reporting Checklist for Authors, Editors, and Reviewers of Meta-analyses of Observational Studies

Reporting of background should include
 Problem definition
 Hypothesis statement
 Description of study outcome(s)
 Type of exposure or intervention used
 Type of study designs used
 Study population
Reporting of search strategy should include
 Qualifications of searchers (eg, librarians and investigators)
 Search strategy, including time period included in the synthesis and keywords
 Effort to include all available studies, including contact with authors
 Databases and registries searched
 Search software used, name and version, including special features used (eg, explosion)
 Use of hand searching (eg, reference lists of obtained articles)
 List of citations located and those excluded, including justification
 Method of addressing articles published in languages other than English
 Method of handling abstracts and unpublished studies
 Description of any contact with authors
Reporting of methods shoulod include
 Description of relevance or appropriateness of studies assembled for assessing the hypothesis to be tested
 Rationale for the selection and coding of data (eg, sound clinical principles or convenience)
 Documentation of how data were classified and coded (eg, multiple raters, blinding, and interrater reliability)
 Assessment of confounding (eg, comparability of cases and controls in studies where appropriate)
 Assessment of study quality, including blinding of quality assessors; stratification or regression on possible predictors of study results
 Assessment of heterogeneity
 Description of statistical methods (eg, complete description of fixed or random effects models, justification of whether the chosen models account for predictors of study results, dose-response models, or cumulative meta-analysis) in sufficient detail to be replicated
 Provision of appropriate tables and graphics
Reporting of results should include
 Graphic summarizing individual study estimates and overall estimate
 Table giving descriptive information for each study included
 Results of sensitivity testing (eg, subgroup analysis)
 Indication of statistical uncertainty of findings

(*continued*)

Reporting of discussion should include
Quantitative assessment of bias (eg, publication bias)
Justification for exclusion (eg, exclusion of non-English-language citations)
Assessment of quality of included studies
Reporting of conclusions should include
Consideration of alternative explanations for observed results
Generalization of the conclusions (ie, appropriate for the data presented
and within the domain of the literature review)
Guidelines for future research
Disclosure of funding source

References

Abramson, J. H., and Z. H. Abramson. (2001). *Making Sense of Data*. New York, Oxford University Press.

Allen, I. E., and I. Olkin. (1999). "Estimating time to conduct a meta-analysis from number of citations retrieved." *Journal of the American Medical Association* 282(7): 634–635.

Committee on Environmental Epidemiology and Commission on Life Sciences. (1997). *Environmental Epidemiology: Use of the Gray Literature and Other Data in Environmental Epidemiology*. Washington, DC, National Academy Press.

Data Quality Act, Public Law 106–554; H.R. 5658 (2002).

Egger, M., and G. D. Smith. (1997). "Meta-analysis: Potentials and promise." *British Medical Journal* 315(7119): 1371–1374.

Egger, M., G. D. Smith, et al. (1997). "Meta-analysis: Principles and procedures." *British Medical Journal* 315(7121): 1533–1537.

Egger, M., G. D. Smith, et al. (2001). Rationale, potentials, and promise of systematic reviews. In *Systematic Reviews in Health Care: Meta-analysis in Context*. M. Egger, G. D. Smith, and D. G. Altman, eds. British Medical Journal.

Federal Focus, Inc. (1996). *Principles for Evaluating Epidemiologic Data in Regulatory Risk Assessment*. Washington, DC, Author.

Federal Focus, Inc. (1999). *Epidemiology in Hazard and Risk Assessment*. Washington, DC, Author.

Graham, J. D., Ed. (1995). *The Role of Epidemiology in Regulatory Risk Assessment*. Amsterdam, Elsevier Science.

Last, J. M. (1995). *A Dictionary of Epidemiology*. New York, Oxford University Press.

Light, R. J., and D. B. Pillemer. (1984). *Summing Up: The Science of Reviewing Research*. Cambridge, MA, Harvard University Press.

Stroup, D. F., J. A. Berlin, et al. (2000). "Meta-analysis of observational studies in epidemiology." *JAMA* 283(15): 2008–2012.

Sutton, A. J., S. J. Duval, et al. (2000). "Empirical assessment of effect of publication bias on meta-analyses." *British Medical Journal* 320: 1574–1577.

World Health Organization Working Group. (2000). "Evaluation and use of epidemiological evidence for environmental health risk assessment: WHO guideline document." *Environmental Health Perspectives* 108(10): 997–1002.

9

RISK ASSESSMENT

Steven A. Anderson and Sherri B. Dennis

The relatively new field of food safety risk assessment provides the link by which a broad base of scientific knowledge can be synthesized into a meaningful product, inform regulatory decisions, and reduce food-borne risks. Risk assessment for foods is rooted in the chemical and toxicological risk assessment methodologies developed for environmental risks. The 1983 National Research Council (NRC) publication *Risk Assessment in the Federal Government: Managing the Process*, often referred to as the "Red Book," established a four-part risk assessment paradigm consisting of hazard identification, dose response, exposure assessment, and risk characterization. This approach characterizes a hazard and its consequential risk in a way that can inform risk management decisions.

The 1993 outbreak of *E. coli* O157:H7 associated with undercooked ground beef hamburgers at a fast-food chain in the Pacific Northwest ushered in a shift in emphasis in U.S. food safety from chemical hazards to microbiological hazards. The effects of illnesses from ingestion of microbial pathogens can be more acute and immediate than the hazards posed from exposures to chemicals, such as cancer. Advances in the field of predictive microbiology in the mid-1990s soon showed that it was possible to predict the growth of pathogens in foods and to model human exposures to zoonotic food-borne pathogens (Buchanan and Whiting, 1996). Increased computational capabilities and modeling software facilitated the development of computer models capable of complex calculations and simulations using sophisticated mathematical techniques. In 1998 the U.S. Department of Agriculture (USDA) issued the first U.S. microbial risk assessment for a food-borne pathogen–product combination. This work was shortly followed by other quantitative microbial risk assessments (see table 9-1).

Microbial risk assessment framework and mathematical models provide a means of estimating the likelihood and magnitude of risks such as illness and adverse outcomes. Furthermore, quantitative models offer a means of comparing and identifying optimal risk reduction measures that can inform the regulatory decision-making process, including those that affect global trade issues.

TABLE 9-1   Selected quantitative microbial risk assessments

Pathogen	Product	Reference
Salmonella Enteritidis	Shell eggs and egg products	U.S. Department of Agriculture, Food Safety and Inspection Service (1998) U.S. Department of Agriculture, Food Safety and Inspection Service (2004, revised)
Fluoroquinolone-resistant *Campylobacter*	Chicken	Food and Drug Administration/Center for Veterinary Medicine (2001)
Vibrio parahaemolyticus	Raw oysters	Food and Drug Administration (2001, draft) Food and Drug Administration (2005, revised)
Listeria monocytogenes	Ready-to-eat foods	Department of Health and Human Services, Food and Drug Administration/ U.S. Department of Agriculture, Food Safety and Inspection Services (2001, draft) Department of Health and Human Services, Food and Drug Administration/ U.S. Department of Agriculture, Food Safety and Inspection Services (2003, revised)
E. coli O157:H7	Ground beef	U.S. Department of Agriculture (2001)
Listeria monocytogenes	Deli meats	U.S. Department of Agriculture, Food Safety and Inspection Services (2003)
Enterobacter sakazakii	Infant formula	Food and Agriculture Organization of the United Nations/World Health Organization (2004)
Vibrio vulnificus	Raw oysters	Food and Agriculture Organization of the United Nations/World Health Organization (2005)

Food safety risk assessment has also been tackled by the international community. A microbial risk assessment framework for food safety was developed jointly by the World Health Organization (WHO) and the United Nations Food and Agriculture Organization (FAO) and has been adopted by the Codex Alimentarius Commission, which establishes international food safety standards (World Health Organization, 1999). The structure is similar to the NRC framework, including the elements of hazard identification, hazard characterization (dose response), exposure assessment, and risk characterization. The ad hoc Joint FAO/WHO Expert Meeting on Microbial Risk Assessment has conducted several internationally focused food safety risk assessments, including an assessment of *Listeria monocytogenes* in ready-to-eat foods, *Salmonella* species in broilers and eggs, and *Enterobacter sakazakii* in powdered infant formula.

Problem Formulation and Policy Goals

Risk assessment provides the science-based rationale for decision making and begins as part of the risk management process with the identification of the issue. Basic risk management frameworks used by decision makers generally consist of identification of an issue, analysis and assessment of the risk, identification and evaluation of options, decision, implementation of the decision, and review and evaluation of the decision. This chapter focuses on the first three elements: identification of the issue, assessment of the issue, and the consideration of the various options that lead to a decision being made.

A key part of the initial process of launching a risk assessment is establishing a dialog among the risk managers, risk assessors, and risk communicators to determine what issue or policy will be addressed and the scope of the risk assessment and analyses to be conducted. The specific food safety issue needs to be identified and clearly articulated regarding specific food product(s) and the hazard(s) of interest (e.g., the product–pathogen combinations), the population of interest (e.g., the general population vs. specific at-risk subpopulations such as the elderly or young children), and the end point of concern (e.g., illness, hospitalization, death). The food safety issue may be well known or may be an emerging problem. The goal of the risk assessment must also be defined. Is the goal of the risk assessment to generate a prediction of risk to determine if action should be taken or it is to evaluate appropriate risk reduction options, or both? Risk reduction options could target steps in the food system including farming, processing, manufacturing and preparation and consumer handling.

The type of risk assessment appropriate for a specific risk management problem depends on the question at hand and the availability of data. A risk assessment estimates risk and, in some cases, sources of exposure and quantitative reductions based on various interventions. A safety assessment, on the other hand, provides a verdict of what is "safe" based on the conventions of the analysis. Risk assessments can be either qualitative or quantitative in their description of the likelihood of adverse health effects, depending on the extent of the knowledge available, the complexity of the problem, and the time available to conduct the assessment. If adequate data are available, a quantitative risk assessment may be possible; if fewer data are available, qualitative and data gap analysis may be more appropriate.

In quantitative assessments, the risk is expressed as a mathematical statement of the chance of illness or death after exposure to a specific hazard; it represents the cumulative probabilities of certain events happening and the uncertainty associated with those events. Conversely, qualitative risk assessments use verbal descriptors of risk and severity and often involve the aggregation of expert opinions. The quantitative risk assessment technique depends on the available data and the scope and nature of the questions posed by the risk managers. A quantitative risk assessment requires a substantial commitment of resources and thus is not appropriate when risk managers do not need this level of sophistication to make a decision.

The risk assessment team may include experts on consumption, pathogen prevalence, food processing (if appropriate), dose response, and modeling. A team leader should be identified. Administrative support staff is also needed to provide administrative/clerical assistance such as filing and technical writing expertise. A liaison with regulatory, policy, or risk management experts might also be beneficial.

A Food Safety Risk Assessment Paradigm

A number of risk assessment frameworks have been developed—the frameworks used most often in food safety are derivatives of frameworks developed by the NRC (National Research Council, 1983) and the WHO/FAO (World Health Organization, 1999), both of which contain common elements and describe similar approaches and were developed for environmental or chemical risk assessment. Risk assessment is an analytical synthesis that provides a structured, systemwide approach for estimating the magnitude of a risk. With policy question(s) in hand, the assessment of risk begins. The WHO/FAO framework, used here as illustration, describes risk assessment as a four-step process consisting of hazard identification, hazard characterization (dose response), exposure assessment, and risk characterization (World Health Organization, 1999).

Hazard Identification

Hazard identification describes the relationship between the hazard and adverse outcomes. The sources of the agent and its behavior in the particular food product of interest are described, as well as adverse outcomes that might arise from exposure to an agent. It provides the rationale and available epidemiological evidence that identifies the chemical, biological, or other entity as a hazard. Descriptions of a chemical or toxicological agent might describe the usual types of exposure such as acute or chronic. For a microbial pathogen, the growth, survival, reduction during cooking, and mechanisms of pathogenicity are usually described. Available surveillance data can also be described, including the incidence and prevalence of an agent and perhaps trends of pathogen incidence or occurrence over the last several years. Information may be derived from scientific literature, government reports, and other reliable sources. The types of data that are used to develop estimates of exposure or disease prevalence may include epidemiological data from sources such as monitoring or surveillance, laboratory research, clinical studies, or surveys.

Exposure Assessment

Exposure assessment addresses the prevalence or likelihood of a hazard's presence and the expected quantity of agent that might be present and consumed by an individual. It describes the pathways and possible sources by which the hazard could enter the food production system during farm production, production in processing plants, distribution to consumer, and storage, handling, and cooking by consumer. Exposure and risk arise from failures in processes and process controls—the infection of livestock with a pathogen, a failure in processing that leads to contamination of a food, failures in maintaining refrigeration, cross-contamination, or improper cooking that exposes an individual to infection and illness. The scope of the risk assessment will influence the breadth of the exposure assessment. Thus, a farm-to-table approach would be comprehensive but a processing plant-to-table assessment might focus narrowly on risk factors during manufacturing and handling by consumers.

Rearing and cultivation practices on the farm may determine a hazard's presence in foods, whether they are of human, animal, plant or other origin. Some would argue that interventions to prevent or limit introduction of a hazard on the farm might have the greatest impact on food-borne illnesses. But many factors make the control of pathogens in a farm environment difficult. Hygiene and sanitation practices for facilities, sources and quality of water, types of feed or fertilizer, housing, and equipment may harbor or foster contamination by some hazards or growth of microbial agents. Pathogenic microorganisms can be spread from animal to animal or group to group via poor rearing practices such as failure to adequately clean facilities between flocks or herds of new animals or introduction of pathogens from external sources such as breeder stock, new stock, insects, or vermin. Spread of pathogens among livestock can occur from direct contact between animals, drinking from shared water sources, or eating contaminated feces—chickens are notorious for doing this. Pathogens in animal waste from farms or the wild can find their way into water sources used to grow and process produce. Similarly, high fecal coliform and pathogens can contaminate waters where oysters and other seafood are produced and harvested.

The process of shipping products to facilities for slaughter or processing can pose risks such as increase shedding of pathogens by stressed animals or cross-contamination of other animals or products in the same shipment. Hazards can spread from animal to animal during transportation from shipping conditions, such as cramped pens or cages, or via pathogen-contaminated feces that can smear onto the feathers or hides of livestock in the shipment. Smaller livestock, especially poultry, are often transported in stacked cages with wire flooring that allows feces from upper cages to contaminate the feathers of animals in lower cages, which can spread pathogens to uninfected animals. Although the uninfected animal has little time to acquire infection, the feathers or hide can serve to contaminate slaughterhouse equipment and carcasses during processing.

In addition to contamination prevalence and levels, cross-contamination or the transfer of pathogens from one carcass or surface to others is a key process for exposure. Some risk assessors explicitly model cross-contamination, while others choose not to do so. This is largely because of the limited data on cross-contamination from carcass to carcass and from contact surface to food. Cross-contamination is a major consideration in poultry processing, which involves the simultaneous processing of hundreds of birds in high-throughput defeathering machines and the use of water-filled tanks for scalding and chilling. Large livestock such as cattle and swine are usually processed on a more singular basis, but cross-contamination can occur, to a lesser extent, from using shared equipment for processing. The food contact surfaces in any slaughter or processing plant—processing machinery and tools, tanks used in scalding and chilling processes, packaging machinery, or carcass-to-carcass contact—serve as the most likely vehicles for spreading pathogens among carcasses during processing. Spreading of organisms from one carcass to another effects two mathematical functions of special importance to risk assessors—prevalence and the number of organisms. A heavily contaminated carcass can affect many uncontaminated carcasses that follow it in the queue, reducing the level of pathogens for the primary bird but increasing the overall prevalence of the pathogen for the group of birds. Similarly, any interventions used in processing for pathogen control aimed at reducing contamination may reduce the level of pathogens but may also affect the prevalence, especially if it is a highly effective intervention reducing pathogen load by many orders of magnitude.

Risk assessors often break food processing steps down to several components or modules (e.g., a slaughter plant module) and model the behavior of the pathogen—its increase, reduction, or stability in amount—throughout each of the steps. Extensive data may not be available for each step of processing for a particular type of livestock, although the scientific literature may contain specific research articles with microbial data focusing on a specific step or steps in the process that can be used in the model. Therefore, a risk assessor might solicit expert opinion from regulators, consumer groups, industry or other stakeholders to fill in data gaps to link various components of the model. Robust data at various steps of the model can serve as a guide and a reality check for the modeling outcomes.

A slaughter model for a risk assessment of beef might address the following steps for cattle: stunning, sticking, exsanguination, head removal, dehiding, evisceration, splitting, chilling, washing, fabrication, and packaging of meat cuts for further processing or retail establishments (see figure 9-1). Processes such as dehiding and evisceration, with potential to contaminate the carcass, may be explored and modeled in detail, while processes such as sticking and exsanguination may be given only a cursory examination. Because the digestive and intestinal tract serves as the reservoir for pathogens in an animal, special care is often taken to ensure that the contents of the tract are contained and that feces and other fecal/digestive material do not contact carcasses. In some cattle processing facilities, the rectum may be tied off or sealed early in processing to prevent leakage of potentially contaminated waste before evisceration of the carcass. As part of the process, USDA inspectors inspect each carcass for visible signs of fecal contamination and may remove any contaminated carcasses.

Food preparation hygiene and cooking may have the single greatest impact on the risk of food-borne illness. Properly handled and cooked, foods pose little risk of illness. Of importance to risk assessors are failures in processes such as refrigeration, handling, cooking, and others that might lead to contamination of product and potentially expose a consumer to a hazard. Cross-contamination from contaminated surfaces (i.e., other carcasses, equipment, tabletops, utensils, containers, and hands) during processing or in the consumer kitchen may be an especially important potential source of exposure that is rarely addressed in risk assessments because data sources may be limited or nonexistent.

Maintaining the integrity of refrigeration throughout processing and production through to handling by consumers is an important risk reduction

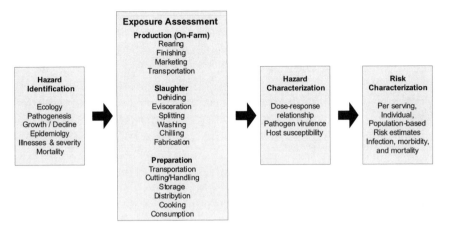

Figure 9-1. Diagram of generic risk assessment process for a food-borne pathogen–product combination for large livestock.

measure. Even when production and processing are tightly controlled, failures in the refrigeration process (i.e., temperature abuse) may sometimes occur and provide an opportunity for the growth of pathogens on contaminated food products. Growth models can be used to predict the changes in the numbers of microorganisms in food over time (Whiting and Buchanan, 2001). Simple estimates of the growth rate assume a linear or exponential relationship between time and the number of organisms. As models become more complex and comprehensive, they include consideration of growth lag phases, competition between microorganisms, and strain differences.

Failure to cook meat completely throughout the product may enable pathogens that are present to survive in or on the product. This is especially important for ground or nonintact products (tenderized meats, etc.). Organisms can be in the center portion of the product and less affected by the effects of heat. Intact meat cuts pose less risk because organisms are largely confined to the outer surfaces and more easily subjected to the killing effects of heating. Thermal inactivation equations are usually used by risk assessors to estimate the combined effects of temperature and time (at a specific temperature) on the $\log_{10}$ or magnitude of reduction on a population of bacteria. A 1 $\log_{10}$ reduction represents a 90% decrease in the bacterial population. The equations are usually generated from laboratory studies of organisms subjected to specific levels of heat and time in a matrix such as microbial broth medium, but reduction studies using the appropriate food matrix are preferred, although not always available.

As discussed in chapter 5 on dietary exposure assessment, survey data quantifying the consumption of specific foods by individuals in the United States are available from two major sources, the National Health and Nutrition Examination Survey (NHANES) conducted by the National Center for Health Statistics and the Consumer Survey for Food Intake by Individuals (CSFII) conducted by the USDA. Beginning in 2002, CSFII and the dietary component of NHANES were merged. In general, the surveys rely on either or both recall of consumption for previous days and the use of prospective food diaries. The surveys use national probability samples to obtain estimates of national consumption patterns, but systematic biases leading to over- or underestimates of consumption are possible because of patterns of reporting and recall. These data can be used to generate a statistical distribution of the amount consumed per eating occasion and used in turn to generate calculations of risk on a per-serving or individual basis. The individual serving data can be combined with data on the frequency of consumption of the food product (amount consumed per week, etc.) to estimate risk on an annual basis for an individual or for a population.

Hazard Characterization

The hazard characterization component is often referred to as dose-response because it defines the relationship between the amount of a pathogen (the dose) and an adverse health effect for individuals and populations (the response). Types of data used to understand dose–response relationships include clinical studies (human volunteer feeding studies), epidemiological and active surveillance studies, animal studies, *in vitro* studies, biomarkers, and expert opinion (World Health Organization/Food and Agriculture Organization of the United Nations, 2003). Data for dose response in humans may be limited or nonexistent, and risk assessors often rely on extrapolation from animal models or surrogate organisms. A complete hazard characterization may also include information on the host, pathogen, and food matrix factors that contribute to the likelihood of an individual becoming ill from exposure to the organism. Pathogen factors include the organism type, strain, and characteristics of virulence and factors that may contribute to its pathogenicity. Host factors include susceptibility of the individual or population to the agent that is a function of age and/or immune state. Children, the elderly, and immunocompromised individuals may be more likely to have adverse events than otherwise healthy individuals. The characteristics of the food matrix (e.g., acidity, salt levels, fat levels) in which a pathogen is transmitted to the host may also influence the dose–response function and whether or not an exposure will lead to disease.

An example dose–response relationship for *Vibrio parahaemolyticus* is shown in figure 9-2. The Beta-Poisson model defines the shape of the dose–response curve, allowing extrapolation from the observed data from human

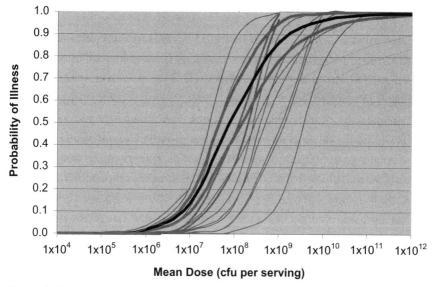

Figure 9-2. Dose–response curve for *Vibrio parahaemolyticus*. The dark line indicates the dose–response curve with the highest weighting (16.5%), and the 20 gray lines represent the dose–response curves with lower weightings (<1% to 13%). Source: Food and Drug Administration (2005).

feeding trials to other (lower) dose levels. The model estimates the probability of the total *V. parahaemolyticus* risk per serving of oysters as a function of the dose. For example, as shown in figure 9-2, the probability of illness is approximately 0.5 for a dose of approximately 100 million colony-forming units (cfu); in other words, for every 100 servings, approximately 50 individuals will become ill.

Risk Characterization

Risk characterization integrates the information from previous steps to derive risk estimates for a population or the risk faced by an individual. The results are expressed as probabilities of potential adverse outcomes for an individual on a per serving basis (e.g., 1 illness per 10,000 servings), individual basis (e.g., chance of food-borne illness is 1/20,000 per year), or population-based risk (e.g., 10 annual illnesses in the United States), which can be expressed as illnesses, treatment by a physician or hospital, hospitalizations, or mortalities arising from exposure to the hazard on an annual basis.

Risk estimates in an assessment are usually expressed using some measure of central tendency—most often as a mean, but outcomes can also be expressed using the median value or 50th percentile. Quantitative risk assessment outcomes should also convey the attendant uncertainty or confidence level, such as 95% confidence interval, or percentiles or the range of values predicted for the outcomes.

A baseline estimate of risk serves as a point of reference to determine the effects of changes of various model parameters on the estimated risk outcomes. Additional modeling for a particular policy or policies and comparing it to the baseline risk estimate the effectiveness of mitigations can be determined by evaluating the reduction in the number or percentage of adverse outcomes such as illnesses, and so on.

Risk mitigation policies can be modeled to explore their effectiveness on the level of risk predicted. Risk mitigation policies may be chosen at a variety of points along the production continuum and may represent additions to steps already present, such as an additional washing of carcasses, to new steps— the interventions should be feasible and reasonable in cost, availability of technology and its adaptation, time spent during production, and effect on the desirability and marketability of the final product.

Modeling Methods

Decisions on the type of model to generate depends on a number of factors, such as the policy need, the time frame for making a decision(s), and the amount of data available. Where the policy question may represent a high-priority regulatory need and data are available, a more complex model may be necessary. When time or resources are limited, a simple, deterministic model may be developed. The rule of thumb in developing a model is that it should be as complex as the question or need, and the available data, time, and resources allow. More complex models have the advantage that they can more accurately convey the uncertainty and variability in the parameters and risk, something that cannot be done with simpler approaches.

The simplest type of risk assessment model is a deterministic model that uses point estimates or single values for parameter estimates. As a hypothetical example, the probability of an animal colonized with *E. coli* O157:H7 entering a processing facility might be 0.1%, and the probability of bacteria from a colonized animal contaminating the carcass during processing might be 0.5%. Therefore, multiplying the probabilities would result in a 0.05% chance of obtaining an *E. coli* O157:H7-contaminated carcass in the facility. To add additional layers of complexity to the simple calculations above, probability point estimates for obtaining a contaminated steak or other meat during processing, probabilities for additional processing and mitigation steps, improper handling, storage, cooking, and so forth, could be added to estimate final probabilities for a consumer obtaining and ingesting an *E. coli* O157:H7-

contaminated piece of meat from the carcass. Additionally, one could add in parameters estimating the amounts of pathogen present on the carcass or piece of meat, reduction in amount of pathogen during cooking or processing steps, amount of product, and organism consumed and a dose–response relationship to estimate the probability of illness from consuming a particular amount of pathogen for an individual, subpopulation, and so on. The risk estimates of deterministic models are expressed as single values for an individual, such as 0.001% chance of illness, or 50 illnesses per 100,000 population expected. The limitation of deterministic models is that a single number as the risk estimate conveys a certain level of precision, when in fact the risk is highly uncertain due to a lack of information used to calculate the risk.

A mechanistic model expresses the underlying processes and behavior of the pathogen(s) and product(s) during each of the various processing and production steps. Mechanistic models are useful because they can reflect the contribution of various steps (e.g., slaughter, washing, chilling, refrigeration, handling, and cooking) during production and postproduction steps on the prevalence and levels of pathogen and can be particularly useful for modeling the impact of mitigations on exposure and the final estimate of risk. Mechanistic models can be either deterministic or stochastic in nature.

A component of the risk assessment model is the dose–response model, which can vary in its complexity, again depending on the amount and type of data available. Mathematical models that have been used to empirically fit dose–response data include Beta-Poisson, Beta-bionomial, Exponential, Weibull-gamma, and Gompertz (Dennis et al., 2002). The extrapolation of these models to new and different conditions or populations is limited. Therefore, there is interest in developing new approaches and capabilities using a more mechanistic approach that will allow inferences in the underlying physiological basis for pathogenicity (Buchanan et al., 2000).

More complex models employ probabilistic methods that use statistical distributions instead of representing parameters as single numbers as in deterministic models. The choice of statistical distributions for a model can vary. Models can be developed from the direct use of data from large data sets. If fewer data are available they can use use probability distribution functions, such as discrete (defined by available data), uniform (defined by a minimum and maximum value), triangular (defined by a minimum, most likely, and maximum value), and gamma. The final risk estimates from a probabilistic model express the result using a measure of central tendency, such as mean or median risk, and the confidence interval about the estimate (e.g., 5th and 95th percentiles). Two important concepts to consider with probabilistic models are variability and uncertainty. Variability is the natural difference of a particular parameter observed across a population for instance body weight, shoe size, and so on. Uncertainty results from limited or a lack of information and factors such as errors in measurement can contribute to the uncertainty in the model. Uncertainty can also arise if the model or type of model used is not a reasonable representation of the processes or issue being examined. Often, no matter how much data are collected, there may be little change in the variability of a parameter because of the natural variation in a population. However, the collection of sufficient additional data can often decrease the underlying uncertainty of a parameter and improve the risk estimate. Simpler models usually address uncertainty and variability together in a single statistical distribution for a parameter, resulting in a one-dimensional model. More complex, two-dimensional models employ separate distributions for uncertainty and variability, which is more mathematically correct but may require additional assumptions by the modeler. Recent versions of software packages used in risk assessment, such as *@Risk* (Palisade Corporation, Ithaca, NY) and *Crystal Ball* (Decisioneering Inc., Denver, CO) provide the capability to generate both one- and two-dimensional models. Again, the modeler, in consultation with other team members, may want to carefully consider the most appropriate approach for their situation.

Stochastic models include an element of chance and may use Monte Carlo methodology. Monte Carlo methods sample from each parameter's distribution to arrive at a single distribution—the sampling process is repeated and thousands of iterations are run, producing a final single, aggregate distribution of the risk estimate. Stochastic approaches are extremely useful and powerful because they reflect the numerous possibilities where chance may play a role in determining the final outcome of risk.

Models are a mathematical representation of a physical, chemical, or biological system and can be entirely theoretical exercises using little or no information derived from real systems, or can incorporate actual data to "anchor" the model and certain parameters. The more data that are used in the generation of the model, the more robust the model and its subsequent risk estimates. Data that may be included in a model include pathogen prevalence in livestock, processing plant product sample data, sampling data of retail product, consumer practices data on handling, hygiene, cooking, and so forth.

Validation is a process by which a simulation model is evaluated for its accuracy in representing a system. All models are, by their nature, incomplete representations of the system they are intended to model, but despite this limitation, some models are useful. Model validation is the process by which the model is evaluated for usefulness. One of the more direct ways microbiological risk assessments are validated is to compare model predictions of illness with epidemiological data. Another way of validating is to compare model predictions with survey data (or other data independent of the data used in the model construction) at intermediate steps to the final prediction.

Model validation is not something that is done at the end of the risk assessment; it involves multiple steps, including the creation of a conceptual model, conversion of the conceptual model into a simulation program, verification of proper translation of model into a computer program, running the simulation program, validation of results of the simulation program, and communication of the results to the risk managers (Law and Kelton, 2000).

Sensitivity analysis is usually conducted as a part of risk characterization and can be accomplished on simple or more complex models. Software packages used in risk assessment such as *@Risk*, *Crystal Ball*, and *Analytica* (Lumina, Los Gatos, CA) provide capabilities to do sensitivity analyses and can generate tornado graphs that rank parameters according to the level of influence on the outcome. During sensitivity analysis, values for parameters are modified and the impact on the risk estimates measured; for example, the impact on the risk estimate from increasing the level of contamination in a plant by a specified increment (e.g., 20% or more). The process is repeated for the remaining parameters, which are changed by a similar increment to estimate which ones have the greatest effect on the risk estimate.

Sensitivity analysis is especially important if assumptions were used in the model because it enables the assessors to explore the impact of the assumptions on the risk estimate. This is a useful means for identifying the key parameters that "drive" the risk or the most influential determiners of risk. Sensitivity analysis can also identify research priorities by highlighting those parameters with the greatest influence on risk where additional research might provide better information and refine the risk estimate to improve its accuracy.

Risk estimates should be analyzed for plausibility and compared to expected outcomes and epidemiological findings from surveillance data or other sources. Limited information about a particular hazard may be available, in which case a hazard identification outlining the available epidemiological and research data and a qualitative risk assessment can be developed that provides a description of data needs and qualitative estimates of relative risks and potential risk reduction measures.

As additional scientific knowledge about the hazard, additional exposure, or dose–response data or improved modeling techniques become available, the assessment and its conclusions may have to be reevaluated or updated. Risk assessments can always be improved, and the uncertainty in the model may be reduced when new data or modeling techniques become available. On the other hand, this makes it difficult to know when to stop and give the results to the risk manager. A general guideline is that the risk assessment should be kept as simple as possible, while providing the risk managers with the information they need to make decisions.

Similarly, the risk assessor often must choose between assumptions or models to use to describe exposure or dose response. The risk management team should be consulted regarding influential choices. They may be able to make all necessary risk management decisions despite this model uncertainty, or they may choose to engage other resources to clarify the choice before proceeding further with the risk assessment (e.g., directed research, expert panels).

Risk Analysis

Risk analysis is a collaborative endeavor orchestrated through the efforts of risk assessment, risk management, and risk communication teams as a means to enhance the scientific basis of regulatory decisions. Each component is unique:

- *Risk assessment* provides information on the extent and characteristics of the risk attributed to a hazard.
- *Risk management* includes the activities undertaken to control the hazard.
- *Risk communication* involves an exchange of information and opinion concerning risk and risk-related factors among the risk assessors, risk managers, and other interested parties.

Risk assessment is one tool that managers can use to help solve a risk management problem or issue. The questions that risk managers must answer are different from those that risk assessors are asked to answer. An example risk management problem is how should the federal government manage the risk of contracting listeriosis from eating ready-to-eat (RTE) foods served in restaurants? In the case of the example of listeriosis, the risk management team might pose questions to the risk assessor, such as what is the exposure to *Listeria monocytogenes* from consuming RTE foods in restaurants, and what is the likelihood of pregnant women contracting listeriosis from eating RTE foods in restaurants.

Risk assessment should be conducted in an iterative manner that allows refinement of the risk assessment question(s), key assumptions, and data used in the model. Stakeholders, including consumer groups, industry, and other government agencies, should be identified early in the process, and communication with them should occur frequently during the assessment. Moreover, the risk assessment document and the process used must be transparent. All assumptions, data, and decisions that affect the risk assessment conclusions and risk management actions should be clearly documented and shared with interested parties.

Key elements of successful risk analyses are a clear understanding of the questions to be addressed by the risk assessors, and a wide acceptance of the assumptions used in risk modeling. Communication of the questions to be addressed often involves an initial dialogue and framing of the issues, followed by clarification and elaboration once screening-level risk analysis has been carried out. By focusing on the dialog among the risk assessor, risk manager, and risk communicator, the risk assessment may be designed to evaluate the effectiveness of a putative action. That is, the risk management question is not just about the magnitude of the anticipated harm—it is also about how we might mitigate the risk.

Additional information on risk analysis including links to risk assessments conducted by U.S. federal agencies and international organizations is available at www.foodrisk.org.

References

Buchanan RL, Whiting RC. Risk assessment and predictive microbiology. Journal of Food Protection. 1996; (suppl):31–36.

Buchanan RL, Smith JL, Long W. Microbial risk assessment: dose-response relations and risk characterization. International Journal of Food Microbiology. 2000 (58):159–172.

Dennis SB, Miliotis MD, Buchanan RL. Hazard characterization/dose response assessment. In: *Microbiological Risk Assessment in Food Processing.* Woodhead Publishing Ltd./CRC Press, Cambridge, England; 2002:77–99.

Department of Health and Human Services, Food and Drug Administration/U.S. Department of Agriculture, Food Safety Inspection Service. Draft Assessment of Relative Risk to Public Health from Food-Borne *Listeria monocytogenes* among Selected Categories of Ready-to-Eat Foods. Federal Register. January 19, 2001 (draft).

Department of Health and Human Services, Food and Drug Administration/U.S. Department of Agriculture, Food and Safety Inspection Services. Quantitative Assessment of Relative Risk to Public Health from Food-Borne *Listeria monocytogenes* among Selected Categories of Ready-to-Eat Foods. Department of Health and Human Services/ U.S. Department of Agriculture, Washington, DC; 2003 (revised).

Food and Agriculture Organization of the United Nations and World Health Organization. Joint FAO/WHO Workshop on *Enterobacter sakazakii* and Other Microorganisms in Powdered Infant Formula. Food and Agriculture Organization of the United Nations (Rome, Italy) and World Health Organization (Geneva, Switzerland); 2004.

Food and Agriculture Organization of the United Nations and World Health Organization. Risk Assessment of *Vibrio vulnificus* in Raw Oysters. Food and Agriculture Organization of the United Nations (Rome, Italy) and World Health Organization (Geneva, Switzerland); 2005.

Food and Drug Administration. Public Health Impact of *Vibrio parahaemolyticus* in Molluscan Shellfish. Rockville, MD: Food and Drug Administration; 2001 (draft).

Food and Drug Administration. Quantitative Risk Assessment on the Public Health Impact of Pathogenic *Vibrio parahaemolyticus* in Raw Oysters. Rockville, MD: Food and Drug Administration; 2005 (revised)

Food and Drug Administration, Center for Veterinary Medicine. Risk Assessment on the Human Health Impact of Fluoroquinolone Resistant *Campylobacter* Associated with the Consumption of Chicken. Rockville, MD: Food and Drug Administration, Center for Veterinary Medicine; 2001.

Law AM, Kelton WD. Building valid, credible, and appropriately detailed simulation models. In: *Simulation Modeling and Analysis* (3rd ed). New York: McGraw Hill, 2000; 264–291.

National Research Council. Risk Assessment in the Federal Government: Managing the Process. National Academy Press, Washington, DC; 1983.

U.S. Department of Agriculture, Food Safety and Inspection Service. *Salmonella* Enteritidis Risk Assessment, Shell Eggs and Egg Products. U.S. Department of Agriculture, Washington, DC; 1998.

U.S. Department of Agriculture, Food Safety and Inspection Service. Draft Risk Assessment of the Public Health Impact of *Escherichia coli* O157:H7 in Ground Beef. U.S. Department of Agriculture, Washington, DC; 2001.

U.S. Department of Agriculture, Food Safety and Inspection Service. Risk Assessment for *Listeria monocytogenes* in Deli Meats. U.S. Department of Agriculture, Food Safety and Inspection Service, Washington, DC; 2003.

U.S. Department of Agriculture, Food Safety and Inspection Service. Draft Risk Assessments of *Salmonella* Enteritidis Shell Eggs and Salmonella spp. in Egg Products. U.S. Department of Agriculture, Food Safety and Inspection Service, Washington, DC; 2004.

Whiting RC, Buchanan, RL. Predictive modeling and risk assessments. In: *Food Microbiology: Fundamentals and Frontiers* (Boyle MP et al., eds; 2nd ed). Washington DC: ASM Press, 2001:813–831.

World Health Organization. Principles and Guidelines for the Conduct of Microbiologic Assessment. CAC/GL-30. World Health Organization, Geneva, Switzerland; 1999.

World Health Organization and the Food and Agricultural Organization of the United Nations. Hazard Characterization for Pathogens in Food and Water Guidelines. Microbiological Risk Assessment Series, No. 3. World Health Organization, Geneva, Switzerland; 2003.

10

FOOD PRODUCTION
AND PROCESSING

James C. Kile

The production and processing of agricultural foods such as canned goods, packaged breads, lunch meats, sausages, chopped beef, frozen meals, and all other possible food items for sale in the supermarket or in the food service industry encompass numerous points at which contaminants may be introduced and pathogens can multiply, if they are present and have not been eliminated. Epidemiologists investigating food-borne disease outbreaks can often trace the cause of the outbreak to some point in the food production process, and public health officials may then intervene in the process to request a recall of the product, inspect and possibly shut down a plant, or in some other way change the process. An understanding of food production and processing is of great value to investigators of food-borne outbreaks, and such investigations, in turn, are used by public health officials to control the outbreak and prevent future outbreaks.

Production

Food products may contain contaminants, or food hazards, defined as any biological, chemical, or physical agent that is reasonably likely to cause illness or injury in the absence of its control. Preharvest production of most food products, whether plant or animal, begins on a farm, orchard, ranch, or other agricultural facility. During preharvest production, both plant and animal products may be naturally or artificially contaminated with these potential hazards. Plant hazards include mycotoxins, agricultural chemicals, microbial pathogens, and metals. Animal hazards include agricultural chemicals, microbial pathogens, metals, and drug residues.

Animal and plant products are exposed to natural hazards such as viruses, bacteria, molds, and parasites found in their environments. The animals raised for food may be inhabited by microbiological fauna that do not cause illness in the animals but could cause illness in humans if the pathogens are not eliminated, controlled, or reduced to an acceptable level by such measures as rinsing, heating, or irradiation. Farm animals can also become infected by pathogens carried by rats, mice, birds, insects, cats, and other animal life found around farms. To address these sources of pathogens, much effort on the farm is directed at monitoring and reducing pathogen levels in farm animals. Several European countries have successfully raised flocks of chickens that are completely free of *Salmonella* and take great pains to protect flocks from infection.

Most countries also put in place programs to maintain and protect animal health. In the United States, the Animal and Plant Health Inspection Service (APHIS) of the U.S. Department of Agriculture (USDA) conducts surveillance and studies of pathogen levels in farm animals. Their National Animal Health Monitoring System was initiated in 1983 and conducts national studies on the health and health management of domestic livestock. Thus, information is available about *Salmonella* and *Campylobacter* on dairy operations, *Salmonella* in U.S. feedlots, and *Salmonella enterica* serotype Enteritidis in egg layers.

When veterinarians study pathogens in living animals, the animal is the patient, and the pathogen level is referred to as prevalence, because it describes the disease prevalence in the population of animals. For epidemiologists focusing on food-borne illness in humans, encountering the veterinary application of the word "prevalence" for the first time can be confusing, because pathogen levels in animals can also be conceptualized as exposure levels (in relation to human beings who are at risk of acquiring the disease). The higher the pathogen levels in animals (and the carcasses, and the meat prepared from the carcasses), the higher the potential exposure levels to humans who consume or handle the meat. This issue of terminology can catch veterinarians, physicians, and policy makers unawares and may even explain some of the difficulties in interpreting data from so many disciplines. Even the word "epidemiology" is used differently by veterinarians responsible for animal health, where the focus is the distribution of disease in animals, rather than in humans. Thus, the APHIS Centers for Epidemiology and Animal Health presents data on prevalence of pathogens in animals, for example, as shown in figure 10-1.

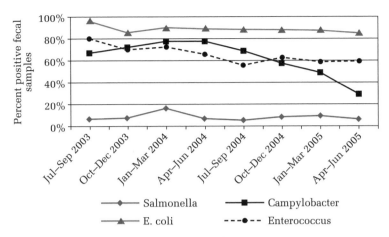

Figure 10-1. Prevalence of enteric organisms in fecal samples in hogs in each quarter over the time period July 2003 through June 2005. Source: Animal and Plant Health Inspection Service Centers for Epidemiology and Animal Health Quarterly Report.

Farm programs to reduce exposure of animals to pathogens can target a specific pathogen and can take different approaches. An example is the effort to reduce levels of trichina (*Trichinella*, a parasite) in pork. In many European countries, each hog is tested to demonstrate that it is free of trichina before it can be sold. In the United States, trichina levels have declined over the past 100 years (see table 10-1). Instead of testing carcasses, the government and industry have cooperated to implement the National Trichinae Certification Program. The program emphasizes good production practices and an auditing process to certify the herd as free of trichina infection risks. The Good Production Practices include use of proper sources of feed, proper preparation and storage of feed, control of rodents, no feeding of wildlife carcasses to swine, cooking of waste food before feeding to swine, disposal of dead animals, general facility hygiene, and the like.

The food fed to animals may have a strong effect on the safety of food eaten by humans. In past decades, pigs acquired trichina by eating garbage; in the 1950s, farmers were encouraged to boil garbage fed to pigs, and modern hog farms no longer rely on garbage in raising pork. Additives fed to animals, such as antibiotics, and pesticide residues consumed by animals also enter the food supply, which raises numerous questions regarding chronic exposure to a range of chemicals. The most dramatic illustration of the role of animal feed in food safety is the example of bovine spongiform encephalopathy (BSE), or "mad cow" disease. The BSE prion infects neurological tissue, particularly the cow's brain, causing a spongelike texture and degeneration of the brain. It is also found in the spinal cord and other areas of the infected animal. The agent

TABLE 10-1 Prevalence of *Trichinella spiralis* infection in pigs in the United States

Year	Percent positive	Number tested	Comments
1898–1906	1.41	8 million	Slaughter testing
1933–1937	0.95	13,000	Grain/forage fed
	0.55	1,987	Fed cooked garbage
	5.7	10,500	Fed uncooked garbage
1948–1952	0.63	3,031	Grain fed
	11.21	1,328	Garbage fed
1961–1965	0.12	9,495	Grain-fed market hogs
	0.22	6,881	Grain-fed breeders
	2.6	5,041	Fed cooked garbage
1966–1970	0.125	22,451	All hogs/national survey
	0.51	590	Garbage-fed hogs
1983–1984	0.73	5,315	New England slaughter samples
	0.58	33,482	Mid-Atlantic slaughter samples
1990	0.16	3,048	APHIS National Swine Survey
1994–1995	0.47	2,132	New England farm samples
	0.26	1,946	Mid-Atlantic farm samples
1995	0.013	7,987	APHIS National Swine Survey
1996	0	221,123	Midwestern market hogs

Source: Trichinae: Pork Facts—Food Quality and Safety, H. Ray Gamble, USDA, Animal and Plant Inspection Service, Beltsville, MD 2001.

remains pathogenic even after exposure to heat through cooking or processing. For many years, cattle parts, including bones, spinal cords, and brains, were mixed into the feed given to animals, including cattle. This allowed the prion to be transmitted to new generations of cattle, dispersing the pathogen more widely, and contaminating the meat supply in many European countries, including England. Unfortunately, 129 human cases between 1996 and 2002 were diagnosed with neurological disease (variant Creutzfeldt-Jacob disease) in Europe and North America before the relationship between "mad cow," animal feed, and disease in humans was understood. Neurological tissue is no longer fed to animals and care is taken in slaughter to reduce the chances of neurological tissue mixing with the meat to be eaten by humans. Measures regarding mammalian proteins fed to cattle vary around the world and have changed as information about the disease is gained. The consumer is unable to take any action (e.g., thorough cooking) because heat does not deactivate the agent, so consumers rely on precautions taken at the farm, slaughterhouse, and animal feed producers.

In addition to feeding practices, the water supply on farms can be another source of contamination leading to food-borne outbreaks. Fruits and vegetables can readily carry pathogens from farm to consumer, and since they may be eaten raw, without any cooking, food-borne outbreaks have been linked to on-the-farm contamination of cantaloupes, raspberries, lettuce, scallions, tomatoes, spinach, and other produce.

After food has been harvested, much of it will be transported in some manner to facilities for processing. Transportation may occur in liquid bulk-tank trucks such as those used for milk, open-bed trucks hauling apples in crates, or livestock trailers hauling cattle or swine. When transporting live animals, factors associated with transportation, such as stress, may increase the shedding of pathogenic organisms, thereby increasing the possibility of contamination during meat slaughter. When transporting plant products, bruising, exposure to the elements, and other factors may predispose them to acquire additional hazards.

Processing

By preventing, controlling, or reducing to an acceptable level during production, fewer of these hazards will follow the food to processing, storage, preparation, and consumption. Food processing occurs after food products are harvested from a farm or other production facility and transported to another facility for additional steps in preparing the food item for consumption. This could include turning apples into cider, milk into cheese, corn into a microwaveable dinner, or cattle into steaks and may require only a few steps in a small building or more complex processes conducted in several separate buildings, requiring thousands of steps.

Food processing is the act of taking raw agricultural goods and turning them into food products. It includes the slaughter and butchering of animals, canning and preserving of fruits and vegetables, grinding grain, and the combination of foods into products ranging from frozen pizza and lunch meats to packaged prewashed lettuce, and everything between. Each food product requires its own process and machinery and poses a unique set of food safety challenges. The food-processing industries employ a wide range of workers with varying levels of skills and training. Slaughterers, meatpackers, cutters, and trimmers usually work at different points along an assembly line, using knives, cleavers, saws, trimmers, and grinders. Some of the equipment is large and complex (e.g., mechanical meat separators), some are small and simple (e.g., trimming knives) and involve rapid, repetitive motions. Other food processing occupations include batchmakers (mixing ingredients on a large scale) according to recipes; machine operators and tenders who work with cooking vats, deep fryers, pressure cookers, kettles, and boilers, again, on a large scale; roasting, baking, and drying operators who may use hearth ovens, kiln driers, roasters, steam ovens, and vacuum drying equipment.

A major reason that we process food is to eliminate the pathogens and to prevent introduction of other pathogens. Elimination (or reduction) can be achieved by an act as simple as rinsing or as complex as irradiation; introduction of pathogens is prevented by packaging and sealing of a pathogen-free product in glass jars, metal cans, or plastic or paper wrappings that are approved for use with food and that provide a barrier between the food and the environment. Many other measures are taken, including use of salt and acids such as lemon juice or vinegar, to discourage microbial growth, and other food additives, preservatives, stabilizers, and emulsifiers. Heating, pasteurization, sterilization, refrigeration, and freezing slow or stop growth, and drying deprives microbes of water needed for growth.

Clearly, thought must be given to each step along the way, to every ingredient, to every tool or utensil that comes in contact with food, and to training all workers involved with the process. In addition, the facility itself requires attention—the design of the facility should not allow dirt, liquids, mold, or other contaminants to fall from ceilings, overhead cat walks, or ventilation systems. Water and cleansers used to clean the plant must not contain hazards, pests must be controlled, and appropriate plans for waste disposal, warehousing, and storage must be developed and maintained. Thought is given to the floor slope, materials used in walls and ceilings, surface treatments, and coatings.

While it is reassuring that much thought has been given to these many issues, the potential for error at any one point is great. Motor oils from broken or malfunctioning meat grinding machines have been known to contaminate ground meat products and cause outbreaks of illness, cooling systems have dripped bacteria-contaminated liquids into packaged lunch meats, and so on— fortunately these errors are usually caught quickly.

As with food production, biological, chemical, or physical hazards that may be introduced during food processing must be eliminated, controlled, or reduced to an acceptable level as it is being processed. During processing, hazards include environmental contamination of products with pathogens in the establishment, such as equipment contaminated with *Listeria monocytogenes*, cross-contamination from one piece of equipment to another or from one contaminated poultry carcass to another, or contamination from storage areas infested with rodents or insects.

Even after processing, products are transported to wholesale and retail outlets, to groceries and restaurants, to cafeterias and schools, and even to homes. Most food is packaged in some manner, in containers for liquids, vacuum packaging for meats, cartons for eggs, or covered trays in boxes for frozen foods. Exposure to hazards is less likely but still possible. During transportation and storage, food products are again exposed to both natural and artificial hazards.

Process Control Systems: Hazard Analysis and Critical Control Points

Process control is a systems approach to ensuring the quality of products or services (Surak and Cawley 2006). A system is a series of steps required to produce a product or service. In process control systems, actions are taken to modify the process itself (rather than the product), during any of a number of steps (critical control points) in the process, to ensure quality of the product. Process control systems are used in many industries, including the automobile, electronic, paint, chemical processing, lumber industries, and food industries, to produce a quality product with minimal defects or, in the case of food, minimal hazards.

Hazard Analysis and Critical Control Points (HACCP) is one type of process control system that has received a great amount of attention. The National Advisory Committee on Microbiological Criteria for Foods (NACMCF) defines HACCP as "a management system in which food safety is addressed through the analysis and control of biological, chemical, and physical hazards from raw material production, procurement and handling, to manufacturing, distribution and consumption of the finished product" (National Advisory Committee on Microbiological Criteria for Foods 1997). HACCP is recognized worldwide and has been endorsed by the National Academy of Sciences, the Codex Alimentarius Commission (an international food standard-setting organization), and the NACMCF. HACCP is being adopted throughout the farm-to-table continuum as the best available method under which to produce, process, and prepare food for consumption.

The HACCP system for food safety developed from two major concepts. The first was the total quality management systems introduced during the 1950s and used for many different product manufacturing systems. The second concept was the work that the Pillsbury Company performed in conjunction with the National Aeronautics and Space Administration in the 1960s to introduce control of process systems to the production of safe food for astronauts. By the 1980s, many food companies had adopted the HACCP principles for producing safe food by controlling critical points in the production of that food.

Seven principles serve as the foundation for a HACCP system (box 10-1). The first principle requires the business in question to proactively identify potential hazards that could occur in its processes. Second, one identifies places in the food manufacturing system where the proper control of the operation or step will result in the control of the hazards (critical control points). For each critical control point, the plan includes a structured and well-defined set of activities, including defining the hazard preventing measures, setting limits critical to hazard control, defining monitoring procedures for the food safety methods, defining what to do if the food safety methods are misapplied, keeping

---

BOX 10-1   Principles of the HACCP System

The HACCP system consists of the following seven principles:

Principle 1

Conduct a hazard analysis.

Principle 2

Determine the critical control points (CCP).

Principle 3

Establish critical limit(s) for the CCP.

Principle 4

Establish a system to monitor the control of the CCP.

Principle 5

Establish the corrective action(s) to be taken when monitoring indicates that a CCP is not under control.

Principle 6

Establish verification procedures to confirm that the HACCP system is working effectively.

Principle 7

Establish documentation concerning all procedures and records appropriate to these principles and their application.

Source: FAO/WHO.

---

appropriate records to ensure that methods were applied correctly, and verifying that the system defined for this critical control point is working.

While HACCP is a generic term for an overall approach to quality control, and food safety, in particular, the term "HACCP" has become strongly identified with the introduction of its use in the meat and poultry industries and with the microbial testing for pathogens required by the Pathogen Reduction; Hazard Analysis and Critical Control Point (HACCP) Systems; Final Rule, issued by the USDA in 1996. Among other things, the rule requires meat and poultry slaughter and processing plants to apply HACCP principles to management of their facilities and requires microbial testing of products as part of the implementation. While HACCP principles require the establishment of systems to monitor control of the processes, accompanying regulations require that the monitoring include systematic microbial testing. As HACCP has been incorporated into other sectors of the food industry (e.g., fish and juice), it has also been accompanied by the use of microbial testing to monitor its success, and for many, the two concepts are synonymous.

A successful program for microbial testing depends on many factors: availability of laboratory techniques for the specific food item, testing for the appropriate pathogens, selection of appropriate food samples during production, sufficient number of samples, procedures for handling samples, and data management, analysis, and interpretation of results.

A food processor implementing a HACCP system would develop its plan beginning with the hazard analysis to identify all food safety hazards (biological, chemical, or physical) that are reasonably likely to occur in the production process of a particular food (figure 10-2). Once all hazards have been identified, those steps that are critical to the control, elimination, or reduction of the hazards are determined to be critical control points. An example of a critical control point in a slaughter plant would be a carcass wash system utilizing a chemical to reduce the number of bacteria on beef or hog carcasses.

Next, critical limits are established for the critical control points, with procedures necessary for monitoring and actions to be taken should a deviation occur from a critical limit. For many processes, this will involve the use of statistical process control methods. Then, recordkeeping procedures are developed to establish accountability and to allow for identification of trends during monitoring. Finally, verification procedures are established to assess that the system is working in the manner to which it was designed.

Other examples of critical control points that would eliminate, control, or reduce to an acceptable level an identified hazard include the cooking step for ready-to-eat foods, the refrigeration of processed foods, the use of irradiation, and the testing for antibiotic residues in dairy cow carcasses, or milk bulk tanks. A brief example of how HACCP might work could involve the industry process of making hot dogs, a ready-to-eat food product. In the many steps required to produce a hot dog, only a few will be identified as critical control points. One of these will be the cooking step, in order to eliminate bacteria or viruses present in the product before it is packaged. The cooking temperature allowed will have narrow critical limits: too low, and not all pathogens will be eliminated; too high, and the consistency and taste of the product will be affected. A continuous temperature chart allows for recordkeeping and monitoring of the product, looking for deviations, in this case variations from the allowed critical limits. If any deviations are found, corrective actions are applied, such as recooking a particular lot of undercooked hot dogs. After the

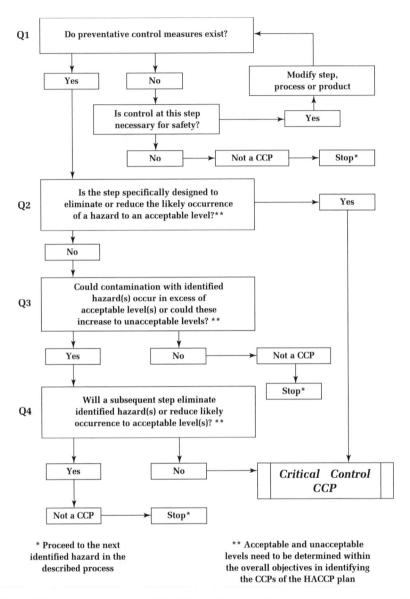

Figure 10-2. Source: Joint FAO/WHO Food Standards Programme Codex Alimentarius Commission (2001).

cooking step, the product is packaged, refrigerated or frozen, and stored. Even in this step, hazards can occur, such as environmental contamination with *Listeria monocytogenes*. Additional critical control points are identified. These and other components of food processing systems must be constantly evaluated to ensure that safe food is being produced.

The food industry and individual establishments continuously conduct analyses for hazard identification and then develop their HACCP plans accordingly to determine that all identified hazards are eliminated, controlled, or reduced or that new hazards are not being introduced, for example, because of a new product or new equipment.

Verifying or evaluating the adequacy of a process control system such as HACCP can be difficult but is necessary in order to determine that the system is working as intended to prevent food-borne illness. However, HACCP is only one part of a number of systems that interconnect in the production of safe food. For instance, most food processors will also have in place good manufacturing practices, standard sanitation operating procedures, microbial testing criteria, and other components. Using some method of systems analysis will help, along with proper monitoring, records, and verification of the critical control points. The entire system of food production, not just the critical control points, should be verified. As public health regulatory agencies, both the USDA's Food Safety and Inspection Service (FSIS) and the USDHHS's Food and Drug Administration (FDA) are required to verify that food processing establishments are meeting regulatory requirements for production of safe food. This includes assessing the food safety systems that establishments have in place, including HACCP.

Figure 10-3 shows four of the primary food production, processing, and preparation systems described above. Each system uses multiple steps to produce food that is safe to consume. All of these systems interact with each other to produce food more safely when they are designed and implemented in an appropriate manner, especially in relation to food handling. Loss of control, even of only one step (an environmental antecedent) within a system, is enough to lead to food-borne illness.

Microbial Testing

Microbial testing is used throughout the food industry to verify that processes successfully reduce or eliminate pathogens from a product. The laboratory test must be reliable, sensitive, and appropriate for the specific food, and sampling frequency should be high enough to assure a high level of confidence that the pathogen is not present (or is present at acceptable levels) throughout the product. This raises technical questions about laboratory procedures and sampling frequency, and the most difficult question of all, what pathogen levels are acceptable, and its corollary, whether any level is acceptable. Many of these questions are addressed by risk assessment (see chapter 9), but accurate risk assessment depends on solid bodies of knowledge; for a world in which pathogens are still being discovered, this is a tall order.

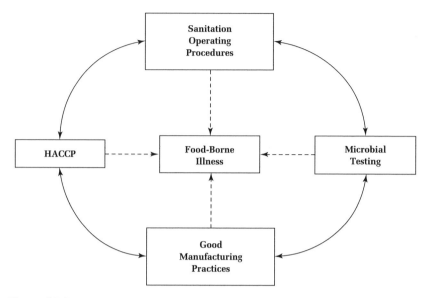

Figure 10-3. Diagrammatic representation of the relationships among food production, processing, and preparation systems (solid lines) and food-borne illness (dashed lines). A breakdown of any step within a system could lead to food-borne illness.

In 1906, when historic food safety legislation in the United States was first passed, microbiology was in its infancy, and microbial testing was not used or required in food safety regulation. This has changed in the century since, but the change has been gradual and, for the most part, recent. Agencies such as FSIS have tested products for pathogens; in 1983, FSIS began testing lunch meats, sausage, and other "ready-to-eat" products for *Salmonella* and in 1987 began testing these products for *Listeria monocytogenes*.

The use of widespread microbial testing as a monitoring end point for food production and processing accompanied the incorporation of HACCP into federal regulatory approaches. In particular, the 1996 FSIS Pathogen Reduction; Hazard Analysis and Critical Control Point (HACCP) Systems; Final Rule requires FSIS to test for *Salmonella* on raw meat and poultry products and requires slaughter plants to test for generic *E. coli* as part of their HACCP plans (adoption of HACCP is also required by the rule). In 2001, the FDA published a rule requiring implementation of HACCP in processing fruit and vegetable juices, again requiring microbial testing of product. The increased incorporation of microbial testing as part of regulatory processes raises scientific and technical questions from many directions. It also has led to the development of databases describing pathogen levels throughout the nation in several industries—data collected for monitoring purposes, but potentially useful in describing national levels as exposures in an epidemiological framework.

Epidemiologists will be asked to assess the association between pathogen levels on a product and incidence of disease in a population to determine acceptable pathogen levels (if there is such a thing) or to estimate the quantitative effect of pathogen levels at a particular point on the farm-to-table continuum on overall incidence rates (see chapter 7).

Contributing Factors and Environmental Antecedents

In order to identify the farm-to-table areas responsible for the introduction of hazards into the food supply, epidemiological investigations must include as much information as possible about all areas of the continuum. Many times data from an investigation provides information regarding ill people or contaminated food items only as far back as food preparation areas, but not back to processing or production. If the food itself was contaminated (i.e., the hazard was not introduced by an ill person during food preparation) the investigation should continue further back.

Whether from a global, agricultural, industrial, regulatory, commercial, or home food-handling practices perspective, there are many contributing factors to the incidence of food-borne illness. The precursors of these contributing factors, environmental antecedents, are variables in the environment that, in the absence of control, may create contributing factors that lead to adverse health outcomes. Five categories of environmental antecedents are applicable from farm-to-table: food and its inherent properties, people, equipment, process, and economics.

The CDC National Center for Environmental Health is conducting research into these "layers" of causation. The CDC researchers hope to describe these layers, determine if there is indeed a causal relationship between these environmental antecedents, the contributing factors, food hazards, and health outcomes. It is hoped that if these underlying systems forces can be better defined and elucidated, patterns may emerge that could be predictive of outbreaks and be used to improve pre- and post-harvest food safety, regulatory inspections, food safety education, and other prevention strategies.

Food production, processing, and consumption are controlled by humans. The human variable as an environmental antecedent may be the most important factor when it comes to food-handling, contributing to food-borne illness in a number of ways. Examples include contaminating apples with pesticides in an orchard, contaminating cattle with feces in a slaughter plant, introducing metal into hamburger during grinding meat in a processing plant, transporting milk to a cheese factory in a contaminated truck, or cross-contaminating during food preparation in a restaurant; humans handle the food.

Helping to identify various food safety issues, Clayton et al. (2002) used social cognitive theory elements to examine the beliefs of food handlers toward food safety. The study identified a number of barriers to implementing safe food-handling practices expressed by the study participants, including lack of time, lack of staff, and lack of resources. Educating the human factor is only a part of the process. Unless people understand the importance of food safety and their role in safe food-handling practices, and are willing to implement what they have learned, the education provided may not be heeded.

Tracebacks in Outbreak Investigations

If the source of contamination is not identified at the point of consumption, but a food has been implicated, outbreak investigators trace the food back to its distributor, processor, and ultimately, the farm on which it was grown, until the source of contamination is identified. Tracebacks are often conducted as part of the epidemiological outbreak investigation but require an additional set of skills that are not part of typical training for epidemiologists. As in the other facets of an outbreak investigation, tracebacks are conducted by persons authorized to investigate the outbreak (municipal, state, or federal authorities, or company management responsible for the site of the outbreak —e.g., a restaurant chain, a school, or hospital might conduct its own traceback investigation). Each organization will have its own set of procedures and guidelines for conducting the traceback investigation (see box 10-2).

The ability to trace a food item back to the farm depends on careful record keeping at each step along the way, and the investigator, working backward, must untangle information about each step to describe the flow of product from the point of error (contamination or failure to eliminate contaminants) to the points of consumption. This, in turn, requires a comprehension of all processes involved, all critical control points, and the ways in which products are produced, delivered, and consumed.

In most traceback investigations, the investigators collect information identifying the product, shipping, and receiving practices, stock rotation and inventory practices, and ordering and product-handling practices. It may begin with a food wrapping or packaging supplied by the consumer (if the consumer still has the package of food thought to have led to the illness—e.g., an egg carton or ice cream container) or supplied by the restaurant or food service establishment (their packages may have been thrown out, but records would be kept describing the delivery of packages and their use on specific days). Figure 10-4 shows food labels that provide information for use in tracebacks.

For example, in the case of illness in ground beef caused by *E. coli* O157:H7, not only do similar pulsed-field gel electrophoresis patterns in human cases

BOX 10-2 Point of Service (POS) Event Information

1. Product Preparation Date/Time (A.M./P.M.):
2. Have there been any reports of illness to the POS?
3. Were any of your employees ill during the two weeks prior to the event?

Outgoing Deliveries to Customers and Incoming Deliveries from Suppliers

1. Can the source of implicated product delivered to customers be tracked precisely by the use of a lot numbering system?
2. How are *customer deliveries* documented or recorded?
3. Are the outgoing delivery records initialed or stamped with the delivery date?
4. How are *supplier deliveries* documented or recorded?
5. Are the records of an incoming shipment initialed or stamped with the receipt date?
6. If the records do not reflect receipt dates, explain how should the recorded dates be adjusted to reflect receipt dates (for outgoing shipping dates and incoming shipment receipts)?
7. Were there any holidays or unusual occurrences that would have affected delivery or receipt dates?
8. What are the transit times from each of the supplier(s) listed above to the current establishment?
9. Are there any transfers of products within the company? How are these handled and documented?

Shipping and Receiving Practices

1. When and how does the firm order new stock?
2. Is there a standard stock "low point" after which the firm orders additional product?
3. What happens if the firm does not have enough product to fill an order?
4. What are the firm's stock rotation practices?
5. Are the stocking practices generally followed at this establishment? When might they be deviated from?
6. Is a stock inventory taken? How often and what time of the day is inventory taken?
7. At what time does this establishment load its deliveries to customers?
8. If inventory is taken, is it taken before or after deliveries for the day are loaded?
9. If inventory is taken, is it taken before or after shipments are received?
10. Did the customer(s) pick up the order or was it delivered?
11. What are suppliers' general delivery times?

(continued)

BOX 10-2 (*continued*)

Product Handling and Storage Practices

1. Does the firm have a standard operating procedure (SOP) and documentation for rejected or returned products?
2. Does the firm have an SOP for disposal of product too old to sell?
3. Is the product prepared, repackaged, and/or handled prior to distribution, service, or sale?
4. How is the customer product loaded?
5. Does the firm mix loads?
6. Is there an SOP for loading?
7. Does the firm have an SOP for truck cleaning or specifications for acceptance of vehicles for loading?
8. Is it clear to the loaders which product should be loaded first?
9. What are the approximate shipping times to the firm(s) who received the implicated product?
10. How is the incoming product handled upon receipt?
11. Do suppliers use any chemical or gas treatment on the product before shipping?

---

and food product allow traceback to suspect ground beef production lots in a processing plant, but further investigation of animal identification systems allow traceback from the processing plant to the feedlot where the animal was fattened and eventually to the producer that raised the infected cattle. Just as processing plants use food production lot numbers and codes on specific days of production, so too can animal producers use animal identification systems to identify animals at birth—a unique number that would follow the animal from the production farm, to the feedlot, and finally to the slaughter plant. This animal's number would be included with other animals and combined into lot numbers for that day's production of ground beef, steaks, and other products. The efficacy and economic viability of other technological solutions to aid traceback are being explored and developed in a number of arenas, including research on animal electronic identification systems (Golan et al. 2004).

Some make a distinction between the traceback investigation and the farm or "source" investigation. One would carry out an investigation on the farm if the traceback leads that far back. Again, the farm environment is complex, and the type of knowledge required to investigate food safety issues on the farm are quite different than that required in investigations in processing plants. The farm investigation may map possible sources of contamination, the slope of the land and drainage, wind-blown sources, and potential flooding or other

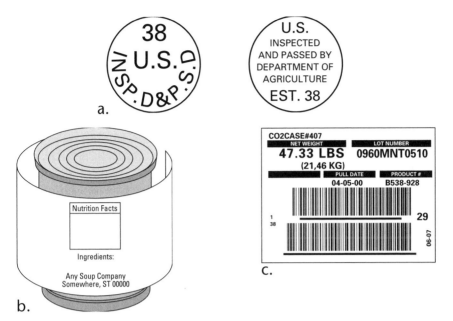

Figure 10-4. Examples of identifying information on packaging used when conducting a traceback investigation. (a) USDA stamps. The meat-processing establishment number is 38; the name and location of the establishment are provided in the FSIS meat and poultry inspection directory. (b) A generic label required under FDA regulations, listing the name and location of the producer. (c) Product label bar code and text giving lot number and the plant coding for the product batch, which provides information on when, where, what, and who produced the product.

weather-related sources of contamination. Investigators will look at manure management to determine whether fresh or composted manure was applied and at what point in the crop growth cycle, water supplies, and the many other factors unique to the farm.

Once the information is gathered, relationships between all sources, distributors, and batches are diagrammed (figure 10-5). Tracebacks and farm investigations help prevent additional illnesses by providing a foundation for recalls of contaminated food remaining in the marketplace and identifying hazardous practices or violations.

Food Recalls

Recalls remove food products implicated in human illness from commerce, thereby preventing additional exposure and illness. Traceback from the contaminated product implicated in human illness to the producer may be required

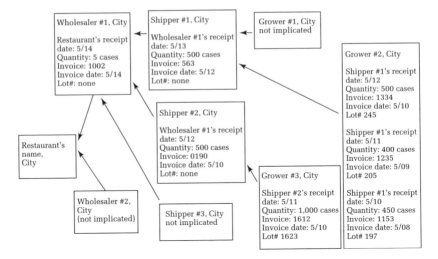

Figure 10-5. Diagram of a hypothetical traceback. Source: Food and Drug Administration (2001).

before issuing a recall of similarly affected product in order to prevent further illnesses or additional outbreaks. However, if product released to commerce is found to contain pathogens during routine microbial testing, some producers may conduct a voluntary recall of the product. Agencies vary in the specifics of their recall authorities. At the federal level, FSIS does not have legal statutory authority to require a recall and can only request the producer initiate a recall. If the producer refuses to initiate a recall, FSIS does have the authority to seize and hold the product until it is determined whether the product contains a hazard to health and, if so, what to do with it (usually it would be destroyed).

For FSIS, then, a food recall is a voluntary action by a manufacturer or distributor to protect the public from products that may cause health problems or possible death. A recall is intended to remove food products from commerce when there is reason to believe that the products may be adulterated or misbranded.

FSIS has three recall stages based on the degree of health risk:

- Class I recalls involve a health hazard situation in which there is a *reasonable* probability that eating the food will cause health problems or death.
- Class II recalls involve a potential health hazard situation in which there is a *remote* probability of adverse health consequences from eating the food.

- Class III recalls involve a situation in which eating the food will not cause adverse health consequences.

The FDA also may issue product recalls if the firm involved is not willing to remove dangerous products from the market without the FDA's written request. If the firm does not recall the product, the FDA can seek legal action, including seizure of available product. FDA guidelines categorize all recalls into one of three classes according to the level of hazard involved:

- Class I recalls are for dangerous or defective products that predictably could cause serious health problems or death. Examples of food products that could fall into this category are a food found to contain botulinal toxin or food with undeclared allergens.
- Class II recalls are for products that might cause a temporary health problem or pose only a slight threat of a serious nature.
- Class III recalls are for products that are unlikely to cause any adverse health reaction but that violate FDA labeling or manufacturing regulations. Examples might be off-taste, color, or leaks in a bottled drink and lack of English labeling in a retail food.

State governments have varying degrees of recall authority for products within their jurisdictions, and various types of recalls are also used internationally, within other countries and across trade boundaries.

Just as establishments that produce food products are required to comply with federal and state laws for food production, federal and state public health agencies are required to comply with laws when considering enforcement actions, such as closing a plant for the production of unsafe food. Federal and state laws allow establishments to have due process of law when a consideration is being made to close a plant for producing food that was not safe. FSIS inspects meat, poultry, and processed egg products and applies the USDA marks of inspection when inspectors are able to determine that products are not adulterated. However, FSIS may temporarily withhold the marks of inspection from specific products, suspend inspection, or withdraw a grant of inspection if a plant is not meeting regulatory requirements. These enforcement actions effectively stop plant operations because the plant can no longer legally apply the USDA mark of inspection to their products. The regulatory aspects of food safety are discussed in greater detail in chapter 13.

From agricultural production and processing to investigating a link between human illness and food product that is injurious to health, epidemiologists must use their knowledge of food production and processing, process control systems, traceback investigation, and federal and state laws applicable to safe food production to assist in the reduction of food-borne illness.

References

Clayton, D. A., C. J. Griffith, et al. (2002). "Food handlers' beliefs and self-reported practices." *International Journal of Environmental Health Research* 12(1): 25–39.

Collaboration in Animal Health and Food Safety Epidemiology. (2005). *CAHFSE Quarterly Report April 1–June 30, 2005*. Collaboration in Animal Health and Food Safety Epidemiology, Animal and Plant Health Inspection Service.

Food and Drug Administration. (2001). *Guide to Traceback of Fresh Fruits and Vegetables Implicated in Epidemiological Investigations*. Washington, D.C.: U.S. Department of Health and Human Services.

FSIS. *Pathogen Reduction; Hazard Analysis and Critical Control Point (HACCP) Systems; Final Rule*; 1996. Published in the Federal Register, 61 (144), July 25, 1996. Available at http://www.fsis.usda.gov/OPPDE/rdad/FRPubs/93-016F.pdf [accessed October 15, 2006].

Golan, E., B. Krissoff, et al. (2004). *Traceability in the US Food Supply: Economic Theory and Industry Studies*. Economic Research Service, U.S. Department of Agriculture.

Joint FAO/WHO Food Standards Programme Codex Alimentarius Commission. (2001). *Basic Texts on Food Hygiene*, 2nd ed. Rome, Italy, Food and Agriculture Organization of the United Nations World Health Organization.

National Advisory Committee on Microbiological Criteria for Foods. (1997). *Hazard Analysis and Critical Control Point Principles and Application Guidelines*. Washington, D.C.: U.S. Department of Health and Human Services and U.S. Department of Agriculture.

Surak, J. G., and J. L. Cawley. (2006). *Implementing Process Control and Continuous Improvement*. Ames, Iowa, Blackwell Publishing.

11

FOOD HANDLING
AND PREPARATION

Charles Higgins

In February 2000, an outbreak of gastroenteritis occurred among banquet attendees at a car dealership in New York (Anderson et al. 2001). The boxed banquet meal was produced by a catering operation in Ohio and distributed to dealerships throughout the United States. Of 742 banquet attendees at 20 dealerships in 13 states, 334 (45%) reported illness. The median age of ill persons was 37 years. Vomiting (61%) and diarrhea (88%) were the predominant symptoms. Univariate analysis of menu items showed an association between illness and consumption of any of four side salads (relative risk = 3.4; 95% confidence interval, 2.33–5.20). *Norovirus* was confirmed by polymerase chain reaction in 29 of 41 patient stools.

A Centers for Disease Control and Prevention (CDC) team investigating the environmental aspects of this outbreak found that none of the employees of the catering operation had extensive knowledge of food safety issues and controls, and no one had any formal training in food safety (Centers for Disease Control and Prevention 2000). No attempt had been made by the establishment to train employees in food safety, and no written information was distributed or posted in the operation. Through observation and interviews, the environmental investigators found that bare-hand contact of ready-to-eat foods was the normal operating procedure in this system. Employees did not demonstrate frequent or correct hand washing. All employees denied having worked while ill; however, many were hourly employees paid at the minimum wage, without sick leave benefits, and were required to bring a doctor's note if they called in sick. Interviews indicated that employees felt financial pressures to work while ill.

Using a cause-and-effect questioning approach, a technique derived from the fishbone diagramming that Dr. Kaoru Ishikawa used in his pioneering work in industrial quality control (Ishikawa 1991), investigators explored the reasons for the loss of control over bare-hand contact with ready-to-eat foods. In this effort to understand the forces that may have shaped this operation, all interview answers led back to the inherent beliefs, attitudes, and business practices of the owner. An obvious lack of interest in or knowledge about food safety issues may have set in motion the sequence of events that led to this outbreak. For this reason, environmental sanitarians emphasize that any attempt to discover the causes of an outbreak associated with food preparation must include an in-depth exploration of the underlying forces that shape each facility.

Food Handling and Preparation Process Controls

As opposed to the rest of the farm to table continuum, food handling and preparation as used here include the handling of foods and/or the combining of commodities in the preparation of meals intended for consumer consumption. These are the last steps that any foods undergo outside of the home, before consumption, and may take place either in a commercial or noncommercial (such as community events) setting. This aspect of the food chain is characterized by an almost endless variety of combinations, menus, culinary approaches, and ethnic or cultural preferences. "Retail food service," as the commercial aspect of this portion of the food chain is often termed, is not categorized in any uniform way, with varying government and industry sources providing differing definitions. Part of the U.S. Food and Drug Administration (FDA) Food Code reads, "Food Establishment means an operation that stores, prepares, packages, serves, vends, or otherwise provides food for human consumption" (Food and Drug Administration 2005). What retail operations have in common is that food is being prepared with the intention of "immediate" consumption by the consumer. While time between preparation and consumption can be quite long in some circumstances, perhaps as long as days or even a week or more, the intent is different from that of production or processing, where foods are expected to be either stored or further prepared. As with food production and processing, process controls can be applied to food handling, to assure food safety. Hazard Analysis and Critical Control Points concepts (see chapter 10) are used at this point by some food preparation companies and facilities; however, most process controls at this level tend to be more informal than those occurring in other portions of the farm-to-table continuum. The commercial or noncommercial kitchens where foods are handled and prepared can be thought of as complex systems, and as systems, they have inputs, process, outputs, feedback mechanisms, and natural "set-points" created by the nature of the underlying system forces (Bertalanffy 1968) (figure 11-1). This systems concept is now in use in the routine food safety inspections that are conducted at food service facilities in the U.S. National Park System (Higgins and Hartfield 2004). Understanding these systems, how they operate, and why they operate the way that they do can also be of value in the environmental portion of a food-borne outbreak investigation. Because kitchens are complex systems, trying to assess them in all of their rich and layered detail during an outbreak investigation, when time is of the essence, can be daunting. Especially during the environmental portion of an outbreak investigation, there is a need for legitimate "shortcuts" to a systems analysis or systems failure evaluation. One approach is suggested by the FDA. The FDA proposes that all foods prepared outside of the home be grouped into one of three categories: foods that are not cooked, foods that are cooked and served, and foods that have complex flows (table 11-1).

Uncooked foods are any of the foods served from a menu or at an event or operation that are never cooked, or commercially prepared or precooked items that are not cooked again at this site, before being served. Foods in this category obviously include various green salads but also include items such as lunchmeats; preprocessed potato and pasta salads; precooked ham, chicken breast, or other meats served without reheating; and breads or desserts not cooked on-site.

Foods that fall into the cook-and-serve category are all of those foods that are cooked on the premises and then served to the consumer without cooling. These foods are characterized by the fact that they transit the temperature danger zone (41–140°F) only once, during the cooking process (transit time refers here to the time that it takes for the internal temperature of a food to change from 41°F to 140°F during cooking; see figure 11-2). Examples of this category include hamburgers, steaks, fish, and other meats that are grilled at the time of an order or just before; and vegetables, rice, or other foods that are cooked and held at hot temperatures but not reused.

Foods with complex flows are all of the foods that are prepared ahead of time and cooled (transiting the danger zone more than once in heating and cooling). Other preparation steps may follow cooling in one or more cycles of preparation. Foods such as soups made from scratch, chili, taco meats, stews, and other items that take time to make are often a part of this process. Many of these food items take too much time to make after an order is placed, necessitating preparing them ahead of service. Preparing complex foods ahead

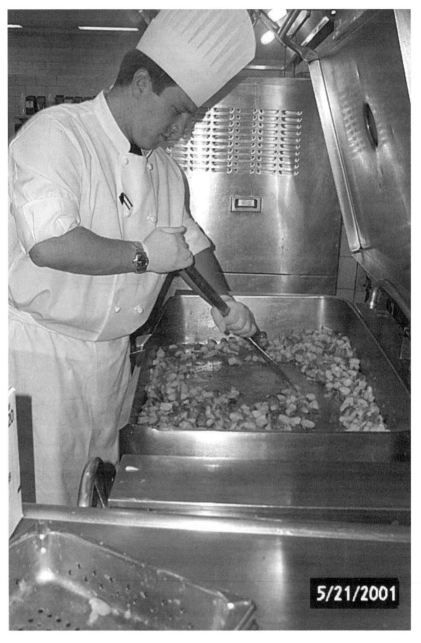

Figure 11-1. Kitchens are complex systems, and every activity in food preparation presents opportunities for contamination.

TABLE 11-1   FDA categorization of foods prepared outside the home

Food	Hazards	Controls
Not cooked	Viruses	Personal hygiene
	Bacteria of low dose	Preventing cross-contamination
Cooked and served	Bacteria of animal origin	Cooking temperatures
Complex flow	Spore-forming bacteria	Rapid cooling
	High-dose bacteria	Cold holdingAdequate reheating

of service also allows commercial kitchens to take advantage of less busy times of the work day when employees are not engaged in meal service. This approach frequently means that these foods, once prepared, must be cooled, stored, and then reheated for service. Other food items that start out as simple cook-and-serve foods may be cooled and reused (such as pasta, rice, meats, or potatoes). This decision switches these foods into the complex category.

These three categories of basic retail processes are useful to an outbreak investigation. In a short period of time, we can establish which foods are in each category, the degree of control an establishment has over each process, and why control is maintained or lost. Not only do all menu items fit into one

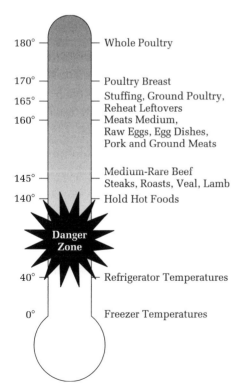

Figure 11-2. An educational tool helping food preparers understand the importance of temperature of food and food safety. Source: CFSAN/FDA.

of these processes, but also this grouping aligns with how most outbreaks occur, with the hazards associated with different foods, with the necessary controls for the inherent hazards, and how operations plan and prepare meals. For example, in most medium to large commercial kitchens, room and equipment layout are arranged around a cook's line (where foods in the cook-and-serve category predominate), an area behind the cook's line called the prep area (where complex flows are concentrated), and a pantry (where food items are most likely to be in a ready-to-eat form). Hazards and outbreak align nicely in these same three areas. Low-dose organisms that do not require time to multiply, such as *Norovirus* or hepatitis A, are the predominant hazard for the pantry area. Organisms, usually of animal origin, that do not produce spores or do not survive cooking are the central threat for the operations taking place at the cook's line. Bacteria that produce spores or that require time to grow to large numbers in order to produce illness take advantage of the processes used in the prep area. Because these hazards of contamination, survival, and growth parallel the design of the facility and the menu, these categories can also be used to organize the environmental portion of an outbreak investigation. A process control evaluation can also be used to organize an environmental investigation for chemical and physical agents, although these agents are less frequently the cause of food-borne outbreaks.

During on outbreak investigation, the environment or system in which the transmission may have occurred can be evaluated using the following steps (see box 11-1). First, separate the menu items or foods served into the three process categories. Then, evaluate the degree of active control this operation has over each process. This control is evaluated by a combination of observation, questions, and measurements. In the real, messy world of food preparation, there is rarely such a thing as "always controlled" or "never controlled." It is highly likely that discussion and observation will reveal varying amounts of control determined by time of day, item, who is involved, and other underlying factors.

Using questions, observations, and measurements, foods that represent typical items in each category or, even better, that are similar to foods that may have a statistical association with the outbreak, should be followed through production. For example, if we are interested in a beef stew, we can start by having the operator explain the process, writing or drawing a flow chart and noting on it all of the attendant context: times, locations of preparation, employees involved, temperatures used, equipment involved, and so forth.

After "mapping" the basic process, measurements and observations can be used to capture key food safety issues at each step. One may measure the final cooking temperature and the final cooling temperature and describe the temperature changes over time. Reheat and hot holding temperatures can be measured, as well as postcooking food handling and possible points of contamination. The end result is a flow chart that has appended to it various data

---

BOX 11-1 System Evaluation Steps

1. Categorize the menu items into three universal process categories
   a. Foods not cooked
   b. Foods cooked and served
   c. Foods that undergo complex preparation
2. Determine the degree of control for each process
3. Investigate root causes for control and/or lack of control

---

indicating the degree of control at each step over critical food safety issues (see figure 11-3).

After determining the degree of control over each process or the process involved in the outbreak, individuals or steps that were important to control or loss of control can be further investigated to determine the environmental antecedents or underlying systems forces that may have led to the loss of control. Environmental antecedents may be categorized as the inherent physical properties of foods (pH, water content), people (knowledge, beliefs, attitudes, culture, supervision), equipment (type, maintenance, operation), process (attributes of specific steps), and economic concerns (profit margins, corporate bonuses or penalties).

As an example, one may consider the underlying variables affecting the cooling of a beef stew. Among the inherent properties of foods, in this case, the beef stew, one would consider the density of the stew, including its water

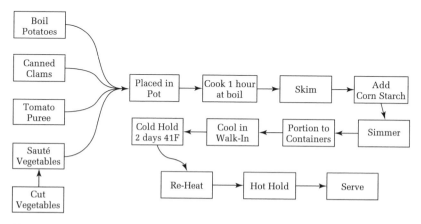

Figure 11-3. An example of a food flow chart showing steps in preparing clam chowder. Key food safety parameters of temperature, time, and handling can be added inside or next to operational boxes to illustrate conditions at those steps.

content, and the viscosity of the stew (affecting the presence or absence of convective currents). Among the variables pertaining to the effects of people, a lack of training or supervision might lead an employee to place the stew in a rapid chill unit but not reset the cycle, turning the rapid chill unit into a common refrigerator, which takes much longer to cool the stew. Furthermore, lack of personal experience with food-borne illness, not having personally "seen" an illness caused by foods, and a low belief level in the risk of food-borne illness might lead an employee to leave the stew on a counter while going off to break or lunch, increasing the time that organisms are at room temperature. Equipment may affect the cooling in many ways. The stew that is placed into a walk-in cooler with inadequate compressor capacity will cool at a slower rate and lead to higher microbial growth rates. Seemingly small factors such as solid shelving in a refrigerator may inhibit the flow of air and decrease the transfer of heat from the pan to the air, again slowing the cooling process. Changes in processes, such as producing the stew on the same day it is consumed, will remove the need to cool it (a process choice can create, modify, or eliminate a hazard). Economics enter into many of the decisions surrounding food handling. The budget may limit training of employees, maintenance on equipment, sick time offered to employees, and so on.

Foods that are not cooked will not have a kill step (exposure to high temperature, freezing, or other factor that destroys pathogens) or opportunity to reduce organisms once present, and the mere contamination of an item can create a pathway. Foods at retail can become contaminated from two sources, people and other objects (foods, equipment, and surfaces); thus, two "firewalls" must be maintained throughout the operation in order to prevent contamination. The first firewall requires the separation of foods that will receive no further cooking from raw foods of animal origin. Because raw foods of animal origin (eggs, meat, poultry, fish) have high probabilities of being contaminated with pathogens, they must not be allowed to come in contact with foods that will not be cooked. Separation must be maintained along the entire spectrum of preparation, including delivery, storage, handling, display, and service. This separation can take many forms, such as storing raw meats in the refrigerator physically below cooked foods or foods that will not be cooked; the reverse arrangement would allow liquids from meats to drip on foods that will not be cooked. Separation can be maintained by physical spacing, preparing items in different work spaces or on different tables. Sequencing can also be used to separate raw foods of animal origin and foods that are not cooked, for example, preparing salad ingredients before cutting and handling raw meats. In this way, the least contaminated foods are prepared first, and the most likely contaminated foods and foods that will be cooked are prepared later. Washing and disinfecting surfaces, equipment, and hands is another way to preserve this separation.

The second "firewall" is that between people and any contaminant they may carry and the foods they will handle. Maintaining general personal hygiene should be the first and most pervasive intervention to control contamination by people. Of all of the personal hygiene issues, correct hand washing at the appropriate times is the most critical. No less important, but much harder to deal with, are the controls that need to be in place to prevent employees who are ill or shedding infectious pathogens from contaminating foods. Employers in the food service industry often do not provide sick leave for ill workers, who are then faced with the choice of working while ill or missing work and not getting paid. Even though many jurisdictions require operations to have written policies for restricting or excluding ill food handlers, and approaches to handle these situations, many operations do not comply with these requirements. In a number of outbreak investigations, the underlying cause was an ill employee (Daniels et al. 2000; Kimura et al. 2005). As a result, many public health officials concluded that handling foods with bare hands greatly increases the potential for food-borne illness transmission. This resulted in changes to the FDA Food Code (see box 11-2) aimed at eliminating bare-hand contact of ready-to-eat foods. Evaluating control of this issue is primarily achieved by observing employees over time. Employees working with salads or in a pantry area can be followed during the course of 30 minutes or so, noting what they are working with, if and when they wash their hands, and whether or not they use utensils or some other means (including gloves) to avoid the bare-hand contact of foods that are not cooked. Notes from such an observation might look like those in box 11-3. The cook's line is a particularly difficult place in which to control this issue because many raw items, including those of animal origin, are cooked and handled. Often, the same person required to place the raw product onto a cooking surface then handles the cooked product. The potential for cross-contamination is extremely high, and practical solutions hard to find. Multiple products, multiple states of preparation, and multiple tasks make this a likely spot for loss of control. It is also necessary to train employees in the appropriate use and frequent changing of gloves, because the gloves themselves can be a source of cross-contamination.

Cooking temperatures and times that eliminate or reduce pathogens in foods of animal origin are clearly laid out in the FDA Food Code. Given the clarity of information, one might think that achieving control of the possible survival of pathogens during cooking would be consistent. One might also expect that because these outcomes can be fairly easily measured (as opposed to measuring food handling involving complex behavioral controls), food safety regulators and businesses would have long ago identified and corrected any shortcomings. Surprisingly, this is not generally the case. Many regulators and operators short on time do not validate their procedures to see that the methods actually achieve the intended result. Thus, actual cooking

BOX 11-2 The FDA Food Code

The FDA Food Code (Food and Drug Administration 2005) presents a model of regulations for food safety. Its eight chapters and two annexes cover all relevant topics, including the kitchen sink. As an example, chapter 3 is 53 pages and contains eight parts. Part 3-3, Contamination, contains seven subparts, and subpart 301 includes this section with detailed recommendations regarding the prevention of contamination by employees.

3-301 Preventing Contamination by Employees

3-301.11 Preventing Contamination from Hands.
(A) FOOD EMPLOYEES shall wash their hands as specified under § 2-301.12.
(B) Except when washing fruits and vegetables as specified under § 3-302.15 or as specified in ¶ (D) of this section, FOOD EMPLOYEES may not contact exposed, READY-TO-EAT FOOD with their bare hands and shall use suitable UTENSILS such as deli tissue, spatulas, tongs, single-use gloves, or dispensing EQUIPMENT.
(C) FOOD EMPLOYEES shall minimize bare hand and arm contact with exposed FOOD that is not in a READY-TO-EAT form.
(D) FOOD EMPLOYEES not serving a HIGHLY SUSCEPTIBLE POPULATION may contact exposed, READY-TO-EAT FOOD with their bare hands if:
    (1) The PERMIT HOLDER obtains prior APPROVAL from the REGULATORY AUTHORITY;
    (2) Written procedures are maintained in the FOOD ESTABLISHMENT and made available to the REGULATORY AUTHORITY upon request that include:
        (a) For each bare hand contact procedure, a listing of the specific READY-TO-EAT FOODS that are touched by bare hands,
        (b) Diagrams and other information showing that handwashing facilities, installed, located, equipped, and maintained as specified under §§ 5-203.11, 5-204.11, 5-205.11, 6-301.11, 6-301.12, and 6-301.14, are in an easily accessible location and in close proximity to the work station where the bare hand contact procedure is conducted;
    (3) A written EMPLOYEE health policy that details how the FOOD ESTABLISHMENT complies with §§ 2-201.11, 2-201.12, and 2-201.13 including:
        (a) Documentation that FOOD EMPLOYEES and CONDITIONAL EMPLOYEES acknowledge that they are informed to report information about their health and activities as they relate to gastrointestinal symptoms and diseases that are transmittable through FOOD as specified under ¶ 2-201.11(A),

(continued)

(b) Documentation that FOOD EMPLOYEES and CONDITIONAL EMPLOYEES acknowledge their responsibilities as specified under ¶ 2-201.11(E) and (F), and

(c) Documentation that the PERSON IN CHARGE acknowledges the responsibilities as specified under ¶¶ 2-201.11(B), (C) and (D), and §§ 2-201.12 and 2-201.13;

(4) Documentation that FOOD EMPLOYEES acknowledge that they have received training in:

(a) The RISKS of contacting the specific READY-TO-EAT FOODS with bare hands,

(b) Proper handwashing as specified under § 2-301.12,

(c) When to wash their hands as specified under § 2-301.14,

(d) Where to wash their hands as specified under § 2-301.15,

(e) Proper fingernail maintenance as specified under § 2-302.11,

(f) Prohibition of jewelry as specified under § 2-303.11, and

(g) Good hygienic practices as specified under §§2-401.11 and 2-401.12;

(5) Documentation that hands are washed before FOOD preparation and as necessary to prevent cross contamination by FOOD EMPLOYEES as specified under §§ 2-301.11, 2-301.12, 2-301.14, and 2-301.15 during all hours of operation when the specific READY-TO-EAT FOODS are prepared;

(6) Documentation that FOOD EMPLOYEES contacting READY-TO-EAT FOOD with bare hands use two or more of the following control measures to provide additional safeguards to HAZARDS associated with bare hand contact:

(a) Double handwashing,

(b) Nail brushes,

(c) A hand antiseptic after handwashing as specified under § 2-301.16,

(d) Incentive programs such as paid sick leave that assist or encourage FOOD EMPLOYEES not to work when they are ill, or

(e) Other control measures APPROVED by the REGULATORY AUTHORITY; and

(7) Documentation that corrective action is taken when Subparagraphs (D)(1)–(6) of this section are not followed.

3-301.12 Preventing Contamination When Tasting.

A FOOD EMPLOYEE may not use a UTENSIL more than once to taste FOOD that is to be sold or served.

BOX 11-3 Example of Observational Notes

XYZ Establishment, Observational Notes
Handling of Ready to Eat Foods
Prep Kitchen   10:15 A.M.
Employee #1

- Empties waste baskets and takes trash out to dumpster
- Obtains melons from storage and begins cutting (no hand washing, no gloves)
- Puts cut melon in walk-in cooler
- Washes hands in hand sink, puts on gloves
- Obtains cooled chicken breasts from walk-in cooler
- Using gloved hands, debones chicken into bowl
- Takes gloves off and goes to employee dining room for 15 minute break . . .

[Continue making observations to capture full range of duties or as time allows.]

---

often fails to attain the temperature or time required. For example, a kitchen might instruct someone to cook a salmon fillet on the grill at a 350 degree setting for two minutes on a side, without validating that the procedure resulted in the fish reaching the required temperature. Evaluation of this process relies on knowing which foods fall into this category and measuring enough cooking outcomes to make sure that variations across time and commodity, as well as shifts and meals, are all captured. This is essentially a question of sample size. Because we do not know how variable this cooking process is, we have to have enough data to have some confidence that we have captured the range of possible outcomes. Variations occur by the original state of the raw food item (frozen or fresh), type of equipment used (fryers, grills, broiler, ovens, steamers, etc.), the person accomplishing the task (skill, experience, etc.), and time during service (busy or slow). Because it is easy to get in the way on the busy cook's line or to be injured (a lot of hot equipment), these measurements are best taken by someone who is experienced in evaluating a food service operation. An alternative is to ask the manager or the cooks on the line to take measurements and report them to you as they are finished. Because it makes a difference when the temperature is taken, where in the food mass the temperature is measured, and what type of instrument is used to make the measurement, evaluating cooking temperatures is a technical skill that requires experience and training (usually provided by a food scientist).

At the beginning of a process evaluation, one may initially describe only a few food items as belonging in the complex flow category. However, after exploring the system involved, many of the cook–and-serve items may be recategorized under the complex flow listing. Operators frequently forget that foods such as rice, which may initially be thought of as a cook-and-serve item, are often reused or, if prepared in quantity, are prepared ahead of service. Discussion with the staff about the preparation flows and a quick tour of the refrigerators and walk-ins will often correct these misclassifications. Food items where the standard procedure is cook and serve may be switched to a complex flow if the facility is conducting food service that is not standard for them, such as a banquet or off-site catering. Complex food items, or at least a few items that represent these flows, need to be followed from beginning to end in order to obtain information about all the necessary controls. While a great deal of information can be gathered through questioning employees, many variations or omissions of controls occur during these complex preparations and need to be observed directly. The creation of a flow chart with accompanying notes of control can be a very useful and even necessary tool for this category. Figure 11-3 illustrates what such a flow chart might look like for a common complex item.

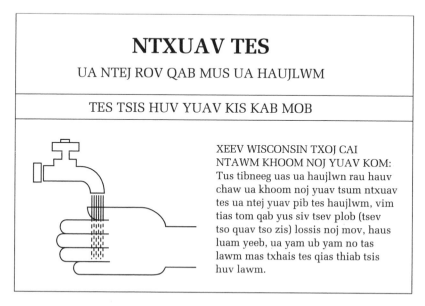

NTXUAV TES

UA NTEJ ROV QAB MUS UA HAUJLWM

TES TSIS HUV YUAV KIS KAB MOB

XEEV WISCONSIN TXOJ CAI NTAWM KHOOM NOJ YUAV KOM: Tus tibneeg uas ua haujlwn rau hauv chaw ua khoom noj yuav tsum ntxuav tes ua ntej yuav pib tes haujlwm, vim tias tom qab yus siv tsev plob (tsev tso quav tso zis) lossis noj mov, haus luam yeeb, ua yam ub yam no tas lawm mas txhais tes qias thiab tsis huv lawm.

Figure 11-4. Food workers are often immigrants who cannot read English; food safety instructions need to be prepared in whatever language is spoken by the food workers. Wisconsin prepared this poster on hand washing for Hmong workers who emigrated from Laos. Source: Wisconsin Department of Agriculture, Trade and Consumer Protection.

Retail Categories

The reader new to this subject may be surprised to realize that no standard categories of retail operations exist and that terminology and definitions vary by locality, state, and government agency. Some of these retail categories, and the characteristics that influence disease transmission, are described here.

Grocery Stores

Grocery stores and supermarkets have changed greatly over the past decades. Within supermarkets, the grocery area has remained central, but add-ons from full-service dining to full-service banking are almost endless. The center of most grocery stores and supermarkets remains the storehouse of packaged and bulk foods and other common household items. If food safety problems happen here (other than the important category of intentional contamination), then it is most likely to be a result of problems on the farm, in production, or during processing. In the storehouse items are mostly protected from contamination by their packaging. They are protected from microbial growth by their physical properties, additives, and preservatives as well as by processing, such as canning.

Other retail departments may surround the grocery department. The bakery is one of the most traditional and common departments. In-store baked items may be made from mix or scratch. Some chains will bake from frozen, partially prepared dough or may offer items baked at central chain bakeries. Some foods may have been purchased from other suppliers. Breads, cakes, cookies, donuts, and desserts are common items prepared at or available from these departments. Some of these items are prepared on-site and are either packaged on-site or not packaged at all. As a result, handling and temperature controls critical to these items may not be as controlled as they might be in a larger process-line–based operation. Some chains, in an effort to appeal to local tastes and interests, may purchase items prepared and baked at small businesses in the community.

If cooking is to be found in a grocery store or supermarket (and there is no in-store sit-down restaurant), then it often takes place in the deli. Besides sliced meats and cheeses, sandwiches, and pickles, many delis produce or provide a large choice of prepared items ranging from twice-baked potatoes to pasta salads, and even whole cooked chickens or meals to go. Many of these items are actually "popout" commercially prepared foods, and the deli only heats or presents them within their displays. However, each store varies, and tracking down individual store procedures is really the only way to make sure. In addition, many stores tweak commercial products by adding extra ingredients to give an item a more customized, local appeal.

The days of having a true, functioning butcher shop within a supermarket are largely gone. Larger stores chains either purchase meats ready for display or package them in central meat processing centers for distribution to individual stores. Some stores may break down larger cuts to smaller ones or may do some meat grinding and packaging. Again, there is variation from site to site. Some meat operations even go so far as to smoke, cook, or otherwise carry out fairly extensive additional processing or preparation. The meat department is a great source of organisms, and if an operation is not run in a controlled way, these organisms can find their way to cooked foods and many other portions of the grocery store or supermarket. Cross-contamination, then, is the key issue in a meat department.

Convenience Stores

Convenience stores come in two basic varieties, those that only sell packaged foods and those that combine features with fast-food outlets, deli operations, and other services in endless combinations. This second category is more likely to produce retail preparation practices that may lead to illness or injury. Because the operational psychology is that of a packed food outlet, those operations that have moved into the preparation of foods may still operate as though they have no real hazards in need of expertise or control. While most cooking processes and products in such stores are simple, ill-informed and poorly trained employees may carelessly handle foods. Difficult processes such as cooling may consist of nothing more than sticking a container in the back of the display cooler or walk-in, without checking to see what temperatures the food may undergo for what times. Hazards may be less controlled in any situation where food preparation is a "secondary" part of a business.

Restaurants

Restaurants cover a wide range of businesses from quick service to full-menu sit-down service. The hallmark of the quick-service restaurants is their reliance on a cook-and-serve process. Foods and menus are engineered so that foods that have been prepared or partially prepared (eliminating time needed for prepping a food for the cooking process, e.g., preformed and frozen hamburger patties) and require only short, simple cooking procedures. In this way, a meal can be served almost immediately after ordering. This reliance on cook-and-serve processes means that hazards are concentrated around two issues, cooking time and temperatures, and handling of the foods after cooking.

Full-menu service generally means that customers sit down and order from a menu that includes a variety of foods requiring a variety of preparation and cooking techniques. These establishments take many forms and depend on different types of commodities and processes according to their culinary goals. What makes these types of retail operations different from quick-service types is the broadening of hazards to include a greater number of food commodities, variation in preparation, complex flows involving longer periods of time, and a wider variety of equipment. Key issues of food safety control in these operations may be extensive, including issues of storage, preparation, cooking, cooling, cold holding, reheating, hot holding, reuse, and handling.

Catering

Combine a full-service restaurant menu with less effective, portable equipment, extend the time from preparation to service, including longer holding times, and you have off-site catering. The hazards associated with off-site catering will most likely be high-dose organisms needing both the right temperature and time in which to grow.

Temporary, backcountry, nonprofit, and community events present a variety of food-handling conditions, from those found at sophisticated commercial operations specializing in outdoor and temporary events, to simple extensions of cooking at home. Depending on the state and local areas, some of these events have been extensively addressed by state or local regulators, and some have not. In some of the largest events, caterers and specialized companies have gained a great deal of expertise in providing foods, under quite innovative and controlled methods, for outdoor or temporary events. In smaller, more community-based events, food may be prepared as a large pot-luck, with the event being simply the additive effort of many home kitchens or prepared on-site as a large outdoor cookout. Regardless of the sophistication of the event, organizers, and food preparation, one of two approaches—pre-event cooking or on-site cooking—is used.

Temporary and Community Events

Because temporary and community events often involve feeding large numbers of people, almost all involve pre-event preparation in order to speed up service during the event. Large volumes of foods may be handled at homes or in food-service establishments. Even the most experienced food preparers may not be ready to protect foods from contamination under these high-volume situations. If pre-event cooking takes place ahead of the event, then the spore-forming bacteria and high-dose organisms needing time and temperature for growth within the food medium may become likely hazards. If the event has taken the opposite approach, cooking everything on-site, survival of pathogens because of hurried cooking is a common risk. Cooking on-site eliminates the lengthy holding of cooked or partially cooked foods, but the rush of getting food out to a large crowd can easily lead to pressures that result in undercooked foods.

Nonstandard or noncommercial foods, containers, and processes are also often found in these events, and when following up on outbreaks associated with community temporary events, standard preparation can never be assumed; all food flows and procedures may need to be reconstructed by interviewing all of the individuals involved. This preparation may have taken place at many locations, under extremely variable processes and conditions, with even the same food items prepared differently by different individuals at different locations and then "assembled" or combined at the event.

Backcountry Events

Hotels, rafting companies, tour operators, professional guides, and others may offer meals in connection with a variety of backcountry activities. From full meals prepared and served on-site during a Grand Canyon rafting adventure to a simple box lunch prepared for a trail ride, these types of operations and foods can vary a great deal. What they all have in common, however, is that food is transported into an outdoor setting. Transportation of foods under these conditions can be a challenge, usually affecting temperature control of potentially hazardous foods. In many respects, these operations have a great deal in common with temporary and community food events. Both types of preparation often occur without the benefit of floors, walls, and ceilings and without the convenience of running water or flush toilets. Innovative solutions to cleaning equipment, utensils, and hands are often necessary, if these issues have been thought through at all by those providing this service.

Nonprofit Events

From shoe-string, inner-city soup kitchens to large, new, community recreation centers, the noncommercial nature of nonprofit operations usually means that the one thing they have in common is a tendency to be run somewhat like a large family kitchen. A wide variety of people may participate in meal preparation, and the foods prepared and served in such facilities may vary extensively. Foods may not always come from commercial sources but may be donated or obtained from local growers; in some states, laws even allow for the donation of wild game or road kill.

Moving Kitchens

Planes, trains, and ships often have moving kitchens, sometimes providing even elegant food preparation at great distances from suppliers. Most of these operations over the years, however, having been the center of much effort by both FDA and the CDC Vessel Sanitation Program, have developed fairly controlled, sometimes, extremely sophisticated operations and procedures. Loss of control in these situations is most likely to result from volume, making handling, cooling, and holding temperatures critical aspects of this type of preparation and service.

Institutional Food Service

Institutional food preparation is almost always one of the most controlled situations, but these operations may also serve the most susceptible populations. Minor loss of control can lead to outbreaks that would not occur elsewhere, so high standards, often tighter than those of other food operations, are frequently followed. These operations are likely to maintain written food production records and measurements of times and temperatures that foods may have been prepared under. Hospitals, especially the larger ones, will tend to be the most sophisticated and supported by resources/staffing, while some nursing homes can be on tight budgets, with almost home-style kitchens and preparation.

Exploring the environmental factors that allowed an outbreak to occur should be a critical aspect of any complete outbreak investigation. Without this step, it becomes difficult if not impossible to translate our investigation results into prevention. If, during an investigation, we can discover where and how the cycles of disease and the cycles of food handling and preparation have intersected, we can begin to formulate intelligent and effective interventions. Understanding the system involved, how it operates, why it functions the way it does, and which variables may be more influential in the final outcome can also help target the epidemiology effort during the investigation. Including an environmental health specialist on an outbreak team will help ensure that the complete triad of agent, host, and environment is fully explored.

With more than a million retail-level food establishments in the United States and a myriad of cuisines and styles of operation, regulation has always been a challenge. Ensuring that regulatory activity is solidly grounded in science and effectively targets real risk factors is an even bigger challenge. Conducting thorough, systems-based environmental investigations as part of an outbreak response may provide us with the data we need to better focus food service inspections nationwide.

References

Anderson, A. D., V. D. Garrett, et al. (2001). "Multistate outbreak of *Norwalk*-like virus gastroenteritis associated with a common caterer." *Am J Epidemiol* 154(11): 1013–1019.

Bertalanffy, L. V. (1968). *General System Theory: Foundations, Development, Applications*. New York, George Braziller.

Centers for Disease Control and Prevention. (2000). Investigating the Environmental Antecedents of a Multi-state Outbreak of Gastroenteritis. Atlanta, GA: Environmental Health Services Branch, Centers for Disease Control and Prevention.

Daniels, N. A., D. A. Bergmire-Sweat, et al. (2000). "A foodborne outbreak of gastroenteritis associated with *Norwalk*-like viruses: first molecular traceback to deli sandwiches contaminated during preparation." *J Infect Dis* 181(4): 1467–1470.

Food and Drug Administration. (2006). Managing Food Safety: A Manual for the Voluntary use of HACCP Principles for Operators of Food Service and Retail Establishments, Department of Health and Human Services, Food and Drug Administration. College Park, MD: U.S. Department of Health and Human Services, Food and Drug Administration.

Food and Drug Administration. (2005). FDA Food Code. College Park, MD: U.S. Department of Health and Human Services, Food and Drug Administration.

Higgins, C. L., and B. S. Hartfield. (2004). "A systems-based food safety evaluation: an experimental approach." *J Environ Health* 67(4): 9–14.

Ishikawa, K. (1991). *Introduction to Quality Control*. Berlin, Springer.

Kimura, A. C., M. S. Palumbo, et al. (2005). "A multi-state outbreak of *Salmonella* serotype Thompson infection from commercially distributed bread contaminated by an ill food handler." *Epidemiol Infect* 133(5): 823–828.

12

THE ECONOMIC CONTEXT

Tanya Roberts

Economists have found that the private marketplace requires inexpensive and good information to operate well. Information about pathogens that could be contaminating food, however, is not readily available to purchasers in the food supply chain. For example, consumers in a restaurant or a supermarket do not know the probability distribution of various pathogens on the food items they are considering purchasing. This creates problems for consumers as well as companies that go to the extra effort to assure safe food. Their competitors have an incentive to cut corners on food safety and sell food at a cheaper price.

Actions by private contractors buying food or regulatory actions can provide these missing economic incentives. For example, in the 1880s European buyers used a microscope to inspect U.S. bacon. When they found the parasite that causes trichinosis, they stopped buying U.S. pork bellies. The value of U.S. meat exports fell by 40% (Roberts, 1983). When the U.S. pork industry requested government aid, Congress responded in 1890 and 1891 with legislation granting official U.S. government inspection of salt pork and bacon when required or requested by any purchaser, seller, or exporter.

Government regulations can also provide economic incentives for all companies in the industry to produce safer food. These economic incentives can be either positive (e.g., requiring all firms to meet a higher food safety standard) or negative (e.g., fines or naming and shaming companies that do not meet requirements). Regulatory tools range from sanitation and testing requirements, inspection, and fines for noncompliance to labels on food suggesting food-handling practices and providing information about food safety performance on a website. Today, the Food Safety and Inspection Service (FSIS) in the U.S. Department of Agriculture (USDA) posts on its website information on meat and poultry slaughter and processing plants that fail residue tests twice in a period of 12 months. Information for pathogens is less well reported. Contamination in meat and poultry products is listed by three categories of plant size, but not by individual plant, on the FSIS website (USDA, 2006).

A critical decision for both food companies and regulators is where to draw the line, that is, what level of food safety to choose as a goal. One indicator of the extent of a food safety problem in the United States is the acute and chronic human illness costs attributable to food-borne pathogens. The USDA's Economic Research Service (ERS) estimates that illness costs at $6.9 billion annually for five pathogens in the U.S. food supply (table 12-1; Crutchfield and Roberts, 2000). The Food and Drug Administration (FDA) estimates that human illness costs of $28.1 annually for nine food-borne pathogens (Raybourne et al., 2003). These high economic costs, for just five of the 250 food-borne pathogens, suggest that too little food safety is produced in the United States today.

The courts play an important role in compensating persons made ill by contaminated food. Awards are minimal, however, because of the information burden. Unless there has been a pathogen test result or a well-characterized outbreak that identifies which food and which pathogen caused the illness, the legal liability system does not work well to penalize sellers of contaminated food. Complex diets, long incubation periods, incomplete lab analyses, and the fact that the food evidence is usually destroyed (because it is eaten) all reduce the

TABLE 12-1 Estimated annual costs associated with selected food-borne pathogens, 2000

Pathogen	Estimated annual food-borne illnesses			Cost (billion 2000 US$)
	Cases	Hospitalizations	Deaths	
Campylobacter species	1,963,141	10,539	99	1.2
*Salmonella**	1,341,873	15,608	553	2.4
E. coli O157	62,458	1,843	52	0.7
Shiga toxin–producing (non-O157) *E. coli*	31,229	921	26	0.3
Listeria monocytogenes	2,493	2,298	499	2.3
Total	3,401,194	31,209	1,229	6.9

Salmonella serotypes other than *Salmonella typhi*.

Source: Crutchfield and Roberts (2000).

chances of successful litigation (Buzby et al., 2001). Occasionally, food markets are dramatically affected by food contamination. Food-borne disease outbreaks and product recalls have forced some U.S. companies to go out of business or dramatically overhaul their food safety practices and controls.

With increasing international trade in fresh produce, seafood, and meat, contamination incidents increasing involve international markets. In the mid-1990s, Guatemalan raspberries imported into the United States were identified as the source of *Cylospora* in epidemiological studies. In December 1997, the FDA issued an alert on Guatemalan raspberries that denied imports into the United States, even though the FDA did not actually observe *Cyclospora* on a Guatemalan raspberry until 2000 (Ho et al., 2002). Since 1997, FDA has become more willing to deny imports on epidemiological evidence (Calvin, 2003). In the United Kingdom, exports of live cattle and beef plummeted to near zero levels as a result of three bovine spongiform encephalopathy (BSE) crises and have not yet recovered (Mathews et al., 2003). BSE concerns also caused beef consumption in the European Union to fall by two million metric tons per year (figure 12-1). One U.S. case of BSE in December 2003 caused U.S. exports of beef to Japan and South Korea to be halted and product in transit to be returned to the United States.

Evolution of HACCP as a Prevention System

In 1962, the International Commission on Microbiological Specifications for Foods (ICMSF), a nonprofit, scientific advisory body, was established to standardize pathogen testing methods for international trade. The ICMSF con-

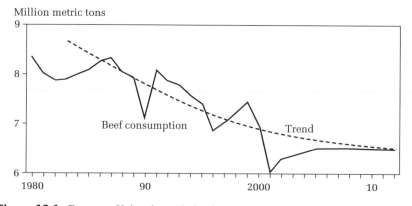

Figure 12-1. European Union domestic beef consumption. Source: Buzby (2003) *International Trade and Food Safety: Economic Theory and Case Studies*, Agricultural Economic Report no. 828, Economic Research Service, United States Department of Agriculture.

cluded, "Testing foods at ports of entry, or end-product testing elsewhere in the food chain, cannot guarantee food safety" (Roberts, 1997). In 1980, a joint ICMSF/World Health Organization meeting examined Hazard Analysis at Critical Control Points (HACCP), developed for the food eaten by astronauts, as a system for controlling pathogens in food. Since the late 1980s, the ICMSF has published several books explaining how food plants can implement a rigorous HACCP system, develop a representative pathogen sampling and testing program, etc. In a pre-HACCP world, when something went wrong, it was not detected and corrective action was not taken. The result was a distribution of pathogen contamination in the food products with perhaps an acceptable mean, but long tails of infrequent, high levels of contamination that are risky and unacceptable. The ICMSF recommended HACCP and its reliance on process control to reduce the variability of food processes (International Commission on Microbiological Specifications for Foods, 1998).

In 1996, FSIS changed the focus of federal regulations from inspection to prevention under the Pathogen Reduction/HACCP (PR/HACCP) regulation. With pathogen performance standards set by FSIS, companies are required to design safety into their food production processes and management practices. HACCP requires detailed knowledge about the characteristics of the food, the microbes of concern, and pathogen controls throughout the food supply chain (Roberts, 1997). Recently, FSIS has strengthened its PR/HACCP requirements for meat and poultry plants (see chapters 10 and 13). The FDA also requires HACCP for seafood and juice products. Further below, a benefit–cost analysis (BCA) of a PR/HACCP regulatory proposal for meat and poultry is presented.

Since the mid-1990s, fast-food companies, large retailers, and importers have started to impose their own HACCP systems and pathogen testing requirements on suppliers (Golan et al., 2004). These savvy buyers act as channel captains and police the actions of firms up and down the food supply chain with food safety audits. Food producers, manufacturers, processors, truckers, and wholesalers selling to these channel captains may garner lucrative contracts, but only if they upgrade their food safety systems to the required levels.

Societal Costs of Food-Borne Illness

All three sectors of the U.S. economy can experience costs or benefits because of changes in the level of food-borne illness. There can be fewer or more persons becoming ill due to eating contaminated food. A change in government food safety regulations, such as PR/HACCP, may either increase or decrease costs to industry and regulators and change the probability of illness to consumers. For this reason, economic analysis is required in major regulations that may have an impact of at least $100 million in 1994 U.S.

dollars (Federal Crop Insurance and Department of Agriculture Reorganization Act of 1994). Industry can change the level of pathogen control required in food purchasing contracts, thereby changing food production practices of suppliers and increasing or decreasing costs (Golan et al., 2004). The following paragraphs discuss the possible economic costs for all three sectors of the economy.

Costs to Individuals/Households   Human illness costs include medical expenses for physician visits, laboratory tests, hospitalization, medications, and ambulance; income or productivity loss for both the ill person and any persons caring for the ill person; indirect costs of illness, for example, travel costs to the hospital, home modifications to accommodate a new disability caused by the food-borne illness, vocational and physical rehabilitation, special educational programs, institutional care, and lost leisure time; and psychological costs, such as pain. Costs can also be estimated for risk-averting behaviors, such as increasing time and effort spent cleaning and cooking or upgrading refrigerator and freezer equipment. Lastly, costs can be estimated for avoiding certain high-risk foods and replacement of these foods with safer but less preferred or more expensive foods.

Industry Costs   This is a diverse set of costs that vary with different public regulations and private policy choices. The impact of new practices to control pathogens in animal production includes changes in the morbidity and mortality of farm animals, changes in the growth rate/feed efficiency and time to market, costs of disposal of contaminated farm animals, new farm practices (age-segregated housing, sterilized feed, etc.), and altered animal transport and marketing patterns (animal identification, feeding/watering).

In the slaughterhouse and processing plant, cost changes can involve carcass trimming and product rework, improved chilling and refrigeration practices, changes in illness among workers handling contaminated animals or products, and changes in meat product spoilage due to pathogen contamination (or an increase in product shelf-life). Improved slaughterhouse procedures can include new hide-washing equipment, knife sterilization, and carcass steam pasteurization equipment. New processing procedures can include increased pathogen tests and possibly new contract purchasing requirements.

Other supply chain practices can be altered, such as product transport using time/temperature indicators. New wholesale/retail practices can involve more pathogen tests, employee training, and other changes in procedures. Some companies will augment HACCP compliance with risk assessment modeling for various links in the food supply chain. Some companies may pay price premiums to suppliers for pathogen-reduced product at each link in the food chain. Other companies may invest in new research to solve pathogen-contamination problems at various links in the food supply chain, such as developing new pasteurization or monitoring equipment, new employee training systems, and/

or new management systems to track, test, and enforce improved food safety practices.

If there is a food-borne disease outbreak associated with a company's products, costs may include herd slaughter, product recall, plant closings and cleanup, regulatory fines, and product liability suits from consumers and other firms. An outbreak may also lead to a reduced product demand because of outbreak. This can alter international trade and be generic to the animal product, that is, affecting all or many of the companies producing a similar food product. To compensate for the bad publicity, both individual companies and industry trade associations may increase pathogen controls and increase advertising or consumer assurances. In instances of large and severe outbreaks, tourism may decrease in that country.

Regulatory and Public Health Sector Costs   Four main types of costs can vary with different regulatory requirements. First, new programs can increase disease surveillance to monitor incidence and severity of human disease by food-borne pathogens or pathogen incidence in the food supply chain from farm to table, or can develop integrated databases for food-borne pathogens (farm to table).

Second, new government surveillance and research programs can lead to identification of new food-borne pathogens causing acute and/or chronic human illnesses, identify high-risk products and production and consumption practices, identify which consumers are at high risk for which pathogens, develop cheaper and faster pathogen tests, and provide new risk assessment models for specific pathogen/food combinations or rank risks in the food chain.

Third, public health costs due to an outbreak can include the costs of investigating outbreak and tracing the sources of contamination and range of exposed persons; testing food products to contain an outbreak; treating persons with food-borne illness or administering preventive medicine, such as serum testing and administration of immunoglobulin for persons exposed to hepatitis A; costs of cleanup; and legal suits to enforce regulations that may have been violated.

Fourth, other regulatory considerations of food-borne disease include concern about the impact on population groups affected (e.g., special concerns for children) and the impact of new regulations on industry costs (e.g., the distributional effects by different regions or by size of company).

Epidemiologic Data Are Critical for Economic Analyses

ERS uses disease–outcome tree models to organize the epidemiological and medical data for their estimates of the human illness costs associated with specific pathogens. Where possible, the outcomes include all the lifetime consequences of acute illness caused by a pathogen. The first piece of data needed is an estimate of the incidence of acute food-borne illness caused by a particular pathogen. The rest of the tree has branches reflecting the major categories of disease outcomes. In its estimates, ERS uses these categories:

- Persons with mild cases of gastroenteritis who do not seek medical attention
- Persons who visit to a doctor's office or the emergency room
- Persons who are hospitalized because of the severity of their illness

For each of these three severity categories, the epidemiological and medical literatures are combed for information about the percentage of total cases that fall into each category as well as the average number of days of illness and the demographic groups that become ill, and information is gathered on the types of medical attention received. National cost data are collected for these medical procedures, medical personnel, drugs, and so forth, in each severity category. Using these data, the ERS calculates the average cost for medical care in the three severity categories. In each severity category, full recovery is possible. Usually, the ERS attributes all the deaths to the hospitalized cases, although this may be a simplification.

Another category of costs, lost productivity, is calculated by multiplying number of days lost from work by the Bureau of Labor Statistics (BLS) average daily wage and the employment percentage for adults. For the premature deaths, ERS uses estimates based on studies of wage differentials for jobs with different levels of health risks. The difference in wages associated with the differences in risk is used to calculate the amount of money workers would be willing to forgo in order to reduce job-related mortality risk. These numbers have been used to calculate the value of a statistical life. Two widely cited surveys of compensating-wage studies place the most reliable empirical results in the range of $1.6 million to $8.5 million (1986 U.S. dollars) (Fisher et al., 1989) and $3 million to $7 million (1990 U.S. dollars) (Viscusi, 1993). ERS researchers chose a midpoint estimate of $5 million (December 1990 U.S. dollars) for their estimates of the cost of a premature death. These estimates for premature death are updated to current dollars using the BLS's Consumer Price Index. To adjust for the age of death, the value of premature death is treated as an annuity paid over the average U.S. lifespan at an interest rate of 3%. Information about the age distribution of deaths is obtained from various sources, depending on the pathogen.

Both the medical costs and productivity losses are summed for each branch of the disease–outcome tree. If there are enough medical and epidemiologic data to estimate the probability and course of disease for sequelae, the ERS may extend the disease–outcome tree model to include them. For example, the common food-borne pathogen *Campylobacter* causes a range of outcomes from diarrhea to paralysis. Since polio has been controlled by vaccination in the United States, Guillain-Barré syndrome (GBS) associated with *Campylobacter* is the most common source of paralysis today. In the disease–outcome tree model for GBS, the ERS divided the GBS cases into two severity categories (see figure 12-2). The age of the patient was a determining factor in the recovery outcome in the most comprehensive study we could find in the medical literature (Sunderrajan and Davenport, 1985).

The ERS's Foodborne Illness Cost Calculator lets users make different assumptions about the incidence of a food-borne disease and different assumptions about valuation measures. This interactive online cost model provides information on the assumptions behind ERS estimates for the cost of food-borne illness. Users can make alternative assumptions and calculate new estimates. The calculator can estimate food-borne illness costs for a state or region or a particular outbreak and can show how cost estimates change under different assumptions about disease incidence, outcome severity, and the level of medical, productivity, and disutility costs.

Disease–outcome-tree models can show the gradual progression of disease over the lifetime of an exposed population. To illustrate this complex sequence of events, the tree in figure 12-3 links exposure to food-borne pathogens to

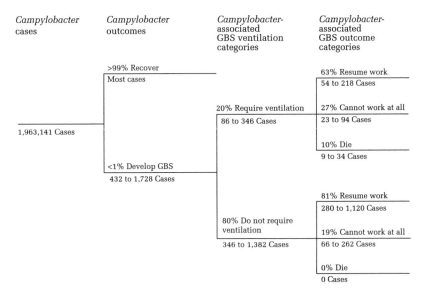

Figure 12-2. Estimated annual U.S. cases and disease outcomes of food-borne *Campylobacter*-associated GBS. Percentages are rounded. Prepared by the USDA ERS. Source: Buzby et al. (1997).

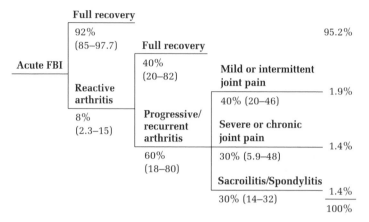

Figure 12-3. Disease outcome tree of arthropathies after exposure to bacterial food-borne pathogens. FBI, food-borne illness. Source: Adapted from Raybourne et al. (2003). Reprinted from Encyclopedia of Food Sciences and Nutrition, Volume 1, Issue 1, R. Raybourne, T. Roberts and K. Williams, "Food Poisoning Economic Implications," pp. 2672–2682, copyright (2003), with permission from Elsevier.

various arthropathies, including arthritis (Raybourne et al., 2003). At the first node of the tree is the estimate of the probability that a person exposed to a food-borne pathogen develops reactive arthritis. At the second node, either full recovery or the possible progression to ongoing arthritis is estimated. The final node characterizes the consequences of lifetime arthritis into three outcomes: (1) mild or intermittent joint pain, (2) severe or chronic joint pain, or (3) sacroiliitis/spondylitis (involving the spine).

Some analysts or policy makers, however, are uncomfortable with assigning monetary values when benefits are human health and safety. To avoid using money as a unit of account, one of the most popular methods is to construct a health index that accounts for changes in both length and quality of life. To calculate quality-adjusted life years (QALY), analysts use individual assessments of health outcomes arrayed on a 0–1 scale, with 0 indicating death and 1 indicating robust good health. With a QALY scale, adverse health outcomes that compromise both lifespan and functional ability are converted to a common unit of account (see, e.g., Food and Drug Administration, 1993). The ERS does not value nonhealth outcomes in its analyses of proposed regulations.

Economic Analyses of Control Options
for a Safer Food Supply

The ERS currently estimates of the costs of food-borne illnesses associated with five pathogens: *Salmonella* (nontyphi), *Campylobacter, Listeria monocytogenes, E. coli* O157:H7, and *Shiga* toxin–producing (non-O157) *E. coli.* The costs are estimated at $6.9 billion each year in medical costs and lost productivity in the U.S. economy (table 12-1).

After the cost of food-borne disease has been estimated for a pathogen or group of pathogens, the reduction in illnesses (and associated costs) can become the public health protection benefits of policy actions. These benefits can then be compared to industry costs to implement the new regulatory policy. The ERS did a BCA of FSIS's proposed PR/HACCP rule (table 12-2). Federally regulated meat and poultry slaughter and processing establishments are required to develop an HACCP plan to identify and control pathogens in their products, meet targets for microbial pathogen reduction, conduct microbial testing to determine compliance with the targets, and establish and follow written sanitary standard operating procedures.

The PR/HACCP regulations for meat and poultry slaughter and processing are designed to control or prevent food contamination by four pathogens: *Campylobacter, E. coli* O157:H7, *Listeria monocytogenes,* and *Salmonella.* Food-borne disease for the first two pathogens is thought to be associated with

TABLE 12-2   Four PR/HACCP scenarios illustrating a range
of net benefits

Scenario	Pathogen control %	Interest rate %	Industry costs	Public health benefits	Annual net benefits
			Present value* evaluated over 20 years (billion 2000 US$)		
Low-range benefits estimate	20	7	1.3–1.5	8.5	6.8–7.2
Mid-range benefits estimate I	50	7	1.3–1.5	21.2	19.7–19.9
Mid-range benefits estimate II	50	3	1.7–2.1	24.3	22.2–22.6
High-range benefits estimate	90	3	1.7–2.1	43.8	41.7–42.1

*Present value is the discounted value of either the stream of costs of the program or the benefits of the program over the 20-year time horizon.

Crutchfield et al. (1997).

raw meat and poultry 75% of the time. Food-borne disease for the other two pathogens is thought to be associated with raw meat and poultry at least 50% of the time. The public health protection benefits come from preventing food-borne diseases caused by these four pathogens. The total case estimates for each of the four pathogens come from Centers for Disease Control and Prevention (Mead et al., 1999). The benefits of preventing illnesses are the avoidance of medical costs and productivity losses for illnesses and premature deaths.

Because the likely reduction in human disease is unknown, the analysis uses different assumptions of a 20% reduction in pathogens (in raw meat and poultry) and in human disease, a 50% reduction, and a 90% reduction (table 12-2). The analysis also uses two interest rates, 3% and 7%, to evaluate the lifetime consequences of exposure to these pathogens and the stream of industry costs. In its analysis, ERS assumes that the benefits of pathogen reduction began in 2000 (when the rule was fully implemented) and extend for 20 years.

Meat and poultry plants are required to develop and implement HACCP plans, follow sanitation standard operating procedures, meet *Salmonella* standards, and conduct generic *E. coli* tests. The costs to the meat and poultry industry include developing HACCP systems and new control procedures, installing new equipment, rearranging product flow, developing new record-keeping, instituting new employee training, and performing more microbial testing. FSIS had estimated these costs to industry and the ERS used these estimates in their BCA.

The ERS found that the PR/HACCP benefits outweigh costs, even for the lowest range of benefits, in combating food-borne diseases caused by four pathogens. With the most conservative assumptions, ERS found that PR/HACCP provided net benefits of $7 billion or more over a 20-year time horizon. When the analysis assumed higher rates of pathogen control and lower interest rates, the present value of the net benefits provided by PR/HACCP were $42 billion.

Conclusions

This chapter has outlined and shown examples of how epidemiological and medical data are critical to the development of disease–outcome tree models. To estimate the medical costs and lost productivity due to an acute food-borne illness, economists need to understand the severity and length of the disease, medical treatments, how much time is lost from work, and the percentage of cases that recovery fully, develop sequellae, or suffer a premature death. All these data are then used to design the disease–outcome tree model for the pathogen of interest.

Once the epidemiological and medical data are gathered and organized into the trees, economists can then proceed to calculate the public health costs of food-borne illness. The ERS focuses on the human illness costs (medical costs and productivity losses). Any reduction in these illness costs is considered a public health protection benefit for the regulatory program being evaluated. In the economic analysis of the PR/HACCP proposed regulation, ERS economists used the BCA model to compare the public health protection benefits to the costs to the meat and poultry industry to comply. This BCA contains three different assumptions about the probability of reducing four target pathogens: 20%, 50%, and 90% reduction in pathogens and in human illness. Even the scenario with the 20% reduction garners net benefits to society, since the public health protection benefit of the 20% reduction in pathogens is greater than the new costs for industry compliance.

A new frontier is integrating epidemiology, economics, and risk assessment. As probabilistic risk assessment (PRA) models for individual pathogens are developed, future models could elegantly estimate the likely risk reduction for the four pathogens HACCP is designed to control (rather than arbitrarily assume a 20%, 50%, or 90% reduction in illness due to the four pathogens in the BCA). The USDA and the U.S. Department of Health and Human Services have built PRA models for several food-borne pathogens.

Another consideration is the short-term versus long-term costs of implementing superior pathogen-control options. As pathogen tests continue to become cheaper, faster, more sensitive, and more reliable, the costs of improved supply chain management systems fall. Why? The new tests improve the accuracy of monitoring pathogens in the supply chain. It is easier to detect the impact of different controls on the growth or decline of pathogens in the relevant food. Consider how pathogen test data from various locations in the plant and in the product can be combined with new data on the performance of existing HACCP programs. This will allow identification of problem locations, continual evaluation of current operating systems and management programs, and evaluation of the success of new changes designed to reduce pathogens in problem areas. In addition, research and development efforts are looking for and evaluating new solutions to improve pathogen control in the slaughterhouse (e.g., steam pasteurization of carcasses) as well on the farm, in transporting animals, in transporting meat, and in case-ready products.

Future research will be better able to quantify the distribution of pathogen reduction into economic analyses (see, e.g., Malcolm et al., 2004). Probabilistic risk assessments (PRAs) are increasingly used by regulatory agencies, and the policy issues are starting to be more formally built into the PRA models as discussed in chapter 9.

References

Buzby J.C., P.D. Frenzen, and B. Rasco. (2001). *Product Liability and Microbial Food-Borne Illness*. Agricultural Economic Report No. 799. Washington, DC: Economic Research Service, U.S. Department of Agriculture.

Buzby J., T. Roberts, and B.M. Allos. (1997). *Estimated Annual Costs of* Campylobacter-*Associated Guillain-Barré Syndrome*. Agricultural Economic Report No. 756. Washington, DC: Economic Research Service, U.S. Department of Agriculture.

Calvin, L. (2003). "Produce, Food Safety, and International Trade." In J.C. Buzby, ed., *International Trade and Food Safety: Economic Theory and Case Studies*, Agricultural Economic Report no. 828. Washington, DC: Economic Research Service, U.S. Department of Agriculture, pages 74–96.

Crutchfield S.R., J.C. Buzby, T. Roberts, M. Ollinger, and C.-T.J. Lin. (1997). *Economic Assessment of Food Safety Regulations: The New Approach to Meat and Poultry Inspection*. Agricultural Economic Report No. 755. Washington, DC: Economic Research Service, U.S. Department of Agriculture.

Crutchfield, S., and T. Roberts. (2000). "Food Safety Efforts Accelerate in the 1990s." *Food Review* 23(3):44–49.

Federal Crop Insurance and Department of Agriculture Reorganization Act of 1994, Public Law 103-54, title 3, section 304.

Fisher, A., L.G. Chestnut, and D.M. Violette. (1989). "The Value of Reducing Risks of Death: A Note on New Empirical Evidence." *Journal of Policy Analysis and Management* 8(1):88–100.

Golan, E., T. Roberts, and M. Ollinger. (2004) "Savvy Buyers Spur Food Safety Innovations." *Amber Waves* (Economic Research Service, U.S. Department of Agriculture) 2(2):22–29.

Ho, A., A. Lopez, M. Eberhart, R. Leveson, B. Finkel, A. da Silva, J. Roberts, P. Orlandi, C. Johnson, and B. Herwalt. (2002). "Outbreak of Cyclosporiasis Associated with Imported Raspberries, Philadelphia, Pennsylvania, 2000." *Emerging Infectious Diseases* 8:783–788.

International Commission on Microbiological Specifications for Foods. (1998). "Potential Application of Risk Assessment Techniques to Microbiological Issues Related to International Trade in Food and Food Products." International Commission on Microbiological Specifications for Foods Working Group on Microbial Risk Assessment. *Journal of Food Protection* 61:1075–1086.

Malcolm, S.A., C.A. Narrod, T. Roberts, and M. Ollinger. (2004). "Evaluating the Economic Effectiveness of Pathogen Reduction Technologies in Cattle Slaughter Plants." *Agribusiness* 20(1):109–123.

Mathews, K.H., Jr., J. Bernstein, and J.C. Buzby. (2003). "International Trade of Meat/Poultry Products and Food Safety Issues." In J.C. Buzby, ed., *International Trade and Food Safety: Economic Theory and Case Studies*. Agricultural Economic Report no. 828. Washington, DC: Economic Research Service, U.S. Department of Agriculture, pages 48–73.

Mead, P.S., L. Slutsker, V. Dietz, L.F. McCaig, J.S. Bresee, C. Shapiro, et al. (1999). "Food-Related Illness and Death in the United States." Emerging Infectious Diseases (5)5:607–625.

Raybourne, R., T. Roberts, K. Williams, and the Arthritis Working Group. (2003). "Food Poisoning (d) Economic Implications." In L. Trugo and P. Finglas, eds., *Encyclopedia of Food Sciences and Nutrition* (10 vols.). Academic Press, Elsevier Science, London, pp. 2672–2682.

Roberts, T. (1983). *Benefit Analysis of Selected Slaughterhouse Meat Inspection Practices*. WP-71. N.C. Project 117: Studies of the Organization and Control of the U.S. Food System, Madison: University of Wisconsin.

Roberts, T., J. Buzby, and E. Lichtenberg. (2003). "Economic Consequences of Food-Borne Hazards." In Ronald H. Schmidt and Gary E. Rodrick, eds., *Food Safety Handbook*. Wiley-Interscience, New York, pp. 89–124.

Roberts, T.A. (1997). "Maximizing the Usefulness of Food Microbiological Research." *Emerging Infectious Diseases* 3(4), 7 pages, web address: http://www.cdc.gov/ncidod/eid/vol3no4/roberts.htm

Sunderrajan, E.V., and J. Davenport. (1985). "The Guillain-Barré Syndrome: Pulmonary-Neurologic Correlations." *Medicine* 64(5):333–341.

United States Department of Agriculture, Food Safety and Inspection Service. (1996). "Pathogen Reduction: Hazard Analysis and Critical Control Point (HACCP) Systems: Final Rule," *Federal Register,* U.S. Government Printing Office: Washington, DC, vol. 61 (July 25) 38806.

United States Department of Agriculture, Food Safety and Inspection Service. (2006). "*Salmonella* Verification Sample Result Reporting: Agency Policy and Use in Public Health Protection," *Federal Register,* US Government Printing Office: Washington, DC, vol. 71 (February 27) 9772.

Viscusi, W.K. (1993). "The Value of Risks to Life and Health." *Journal of Economic Literature* 31:1912–1946.

13

THE REGULATORY ENVIRONMENT

Sean Altekruse

Concerned public health officials, in the midst of an outbreak investigation, often wish to take immediate action by closing a restaurant, closing a farm or manufacturing facility, issuing a recall of product, or warning the public about contaminated foods. These officials quickly find that many layers of government regulation apply to each of these actions. Even activities such as interviewing sick people or discussing information about cases with the media or with other authorities are strictly regulated at the local, state, and national level. After the outbreak has been controlled, pubic health officials may seek to prevent future outbreaks by arguing for a change in regulations in order to regulate the behavior they see most closely linked to the occurrence of food-borne illness. Again, the public health campaigner will encounter multiple layers of government authority—local, state, and federal—as well as various government authorities such as health, transportation, commerce, agriculture, and labor departments that regulate various facets of the farm-to-table continuum. In turn, government action, both in the acute outbreak situation and at the aggregate level of preventing future cases, has increasingly grown to rely on data from epidemiologic investigations, surveillance, and analytical studies to inform policy decisions, most directly, by providing data to use in risk assessments that are part of the federal regulatory process.

Responsibilities for food safety are dispersed vertically from the local through the state to the federal levels and are dispersed horizontally across agencies responsible for health, agriculture, commerce, transportation, and labor. Local, state, and federal governments have varying authorities to pass laws and to enforce those laws through monitoring, inspection, recalls, and closures. Epidemiologic data may be used in some or all of these activities depending on the specific policies of a government agency. Epidemiologic data are most frequently used in an outbreak investigation to guide local decisions to close a restaurant, but they are also used at the federal level to inform policy. Increasingly, epidemiologic data are used in federal decisions regarding product recalls, and epidemiologic data often contribute to risk assessments, which are required for many federal rule-making processes.

State and Local Authorities

State and local authorities have responsibilities for foods that are produced and marketed within their jurisdictions. These agencies work with federal counterparts to implement food safety standards for fish, seafood, milk, and other foods produced within state borders and to inspect restaurants, grocery stores, and other retail food establishments, as well as dairy farms and milk processing plants, grain mills, and food manufacturing plants within local jurisdictions, and have the authority to stop the sale of unsafe food products made or distributed within state borders. Local regulatory agencies include county and municipal authorities. These agencies license local groceries and restaurants and close them for sanitation violations and following outbreaks of infection.

State and local authorities vary in their approaches to food safety. One example is that of Seattle and King County in Washington State, where the focus is on preventing contamination of food by food workers' hands, other foods, or food preparation surfaces and by temperature control, making sure that foods are cooked to temperatures that will kill bacteria. Seattle and King County grant permits to nearly 10,000 food establishments, including restaurants, food and espresso carts, coffee shops, delis, and the fresh food sections of grocery stores and rely on dozens of inspectors to assure that local laws are enforced. Their local laws allow them to close a food establishment for having unacceptable violations on routine inspection, such as sewage backing up in the kitchen or bathroom, no hot water, no running water or electricity, or other imminent health hazards: broken refrigeration, damage caused by accidents or natural disasters, or being linked to a food-borne illness outbreak.

Federal Authorities

In the United States, multiple government agencies have responsibility for the many points on the farm-to-table continuum and contribute to food safety. These include agencies in the Department of Health and Human Services (DHHS) and the Department of Agriculture (USDA), such as the Food and Drug Administration (FDA), the Centers for Disease Prevention and Control (CDC), and the Food Safety and Inspection Service (FSIS) (figure 13-1). Some of these agencies are described below.

Department of Health and Human Services

Food and Drug Administration

The FDA's Center for Food Safety and Applied Nutrition oversees all domestic and imported food sold in interstate commerce except meat and poultry (but including shell eggs) and also oversees bottled water and wine bever-

Food Commodities		Physical and Chemical	
Egg associated salmonellosis		**Pesticide residues**	
Animal disease	APHIS	Sets tolerances for food crops	EPA
Traceback from outbreaks	FDA	Enforces tolerances	FDA*
Continuous egg grading	AMS	**Antimicrobial residues**	
Pasteurization, flock sanitation	FSIS	Sets tolerances for meat and poultry	FDA
Seafood		Enforces tolerances in meat and poultry	FSIS
Safety	FDA	**Food irradiation**	
Voluntary inspection	USDC	Permits irradiation of meat and poultry	FDA
Game animals		Inspects meat and poultry irradiation plants	FSIS
Safety	FDA	*Discretionary enforcement if source not agricultural	
Voluntary inspection	USDA		

Processed Foods	
Pizzas	
Cheese pizza plants	FDA*
Meat pizza plants	FSIS†
Sandwiches	
Open-faced meat or poultry sandwiches	FSIS*
Meat or poultry sandwiches (two slices)	FDA†

*Intermittent inspection
†Daily inspection (also slaughter, meat processing plant)

Figure 13-1. Responsibility for food safety is shared by many agencies at all levels of government. Some of the federal agencies and responsibilities are shown here. AMS, Agricultural Marketing Service (USDA); APHIS, Animal and Plant Health Inspection Service (USDA); FDA, Food and Drug Administration (DHHS); FSIS, Food Safety and Inspection Service (USDA); EPA, U.S. Environmental Protection Agency; USDC, U.S. Department of Commerce.

ages with less than 7% alcohol. In addition, the FDA's Center for Veterinary Medicine has responsibilities for food fed to pets and farm animals. The FDA enforces food safety laws governing domestic and imported food, except meat and poultry, by inspecting food production establishments and food warehouses; collecting and analyzing samples for physical, chemical, and microbial contamination; reviewing safety of food and color additives before marketing; reviewing animal drugs for safety to animals that receive them and humans who eat food produced from the animals; monitoring safety of animal feeds used in food-producing animals; developing model codes and ordinances, guidelines, and interpretations; and working with states to implement them in regulating milk and shellfish and retail food establishments, such as restaurants and grocery stores. A well-known and successful example is the FDA's Food Code, a model for retail outlets and nursing homes and other institutions on how to prepare food to prevent food-borne illness. The Food Code assists food control jurisdictions at all levels of government by providing them with a scientifically sound technical and legal basis for regulating the retail and food service segment of the industry (restaurants and grocery stores and institutions, e.g., nursing homes). Local, state, tribal, and federal regulators use the FDA Food Code as a model to develop or update their own food safety rules and to be consistent with national food regulatory policy.

In 2000, the FDA had about 250 food inspectors to inspect tens of thousands of food operations. Since it is not possible to inspect all of those establishments on even an annual basis, the FDA conducts discretionary inspections based on evidence of need. Regulatory options to remove adulterated foods from the marketplace include voluntary recall by the food manufacturer. In cases of noncompliance with an FDA requested recall, the FDA can initiate a court action to seize a food product or direct the producer to stop manufacturing it (Taylor 1997; Levitt 2001).

Centers for Disease Control and Prevention

The CDC investigates with local, state, and other federal officials sources of food-borne disease outbreaks, maintains a nationwide system of food-borne disease surveillance, and designs and puts in place rapid, electronic systems for reporting food-borne infections. The CDC develops state-of-the-art laboratory techniques for rapid identification of food-borne pathogens, shares these techniques and capabilities with state laboratories, and provides training for local and state food safety personnel.

The CDC provides epidemiologic data used by regulatory agencies to set regulatory strategies and evaluate the effectiveness of their programs. The expanding reliance on epidemiologic data by the FDA and FSIS programs is evident in their collaborations with the CDC and states on surveillance projects such as FoodNet, the National Antimicrobial Resistance Monitoring System

(NARMS; Tollefson et al. 1998) and in laboratory subtyping networks such as PulseNet. These epidemiology-based programs have provided food safety agencies with critical data to estimate the burden of illnesses attributable to specific foods, measure the impact of consumer education campaigns, develop risk assessment models, and formulate policy.

The CDC also conducts food-borne outbreak investigations when invited to do so by states. Often, the FDA and FSIS provide support by testing implicated foods to understand contributory factors of food-borne outbreaks (Tilden et al. 1996; Sobel et al. 2000). Findings from these investigations have been used to support regulatory action and update guidelines to industry. Because of shared interests and complementary expertise, CDC epidemiologists often consult with regulatory officials to gain in-depth knowledge of specific food industries. Similarly, the FDA and FSIS rely on findings from outbreak investigations to guide future sampling and regulatory actions (e.g., banning imports of risky foods, initiating voluntary recalls).

Although the CDC conducts national surveillance for many diseases and maintains centralized databases for those diseases (see chapter 3), the actual authority to report diseases resides with the states. The CDC develops recommendations of diseases that it considers reportable, but each individual state authorizes the reporting of the state data to the CDC. This is an interesting example of a mixture of state authority (disease reporting) with federal responsibilities (analysis of national data).

Department of Agriculture

Food Safety Inspection Service

FSIS seeks to ensure that meat and poultry products are safe, wholesome, and correctly marked, labeled, and packaged if they are transported out of state. FSIS also shares responsibility with the FDA for the safety of intact-shell eggs and processed egg products. States are responsible for the inspection of meat and poultry sold in the state where they are produced, but FSIS monitors the process and will assume responsibility if a state fails to do so. The products regulated by FSIS include domestic and imported meat and poultry and related products, such as meat- or poultry-containing stews, pizzas, and frozen foods and processed egg products (generally liquid, frozen, and dried pasteurized egg products). FSIS enforces food safety laws governing domestic and imported meat and poultry products by inspecting food animals for diseases before and after slaughter and inspecting meat and poultry slaughter and processing plants as well as meat, poultry and egg products. For every animal carcass destined for human consumption, FSIS requires a critical inspection by touch, feel, and smell, a process referred to as organoleptic inspection. Daily inspection is also required in food operations that manufacture food products containing meat. To meet these requirements, at the turn of the millennium, FSIS employs approximately 7,600 inspectors in 6,500 establishments across the nation. Establishments that produce adulterated meat or poultry products are subject to recall. Under extreme circumstances, FSIS can withdraw the mark of inspection, halting interstate commerce (Carr and Lu 1998).

It is interesting to note that in some situations states perform the inspection responsibilities. State meat and poultry inspection (MPI) programs operate under a cooperative agreement with FSIS and enforce requirements "at least equal to" those imposed under the Federal Meat Inspection Act and the Poultry Products Inspection Act. About 2,100 meat and poultry establishments (which are generally small) are inspected under state MPI programs. In the early years of the twenty-first century, FSIS provided approximately $43 million annually to support the 28 state MPI programs currently operating, and provides training and guidance. Establishments have the option to apply for federal or state inspection. However, product produced under state inspection is limited to intrastate commerce. FSIS continually reassesses the criteria by which it evaluates state MPI programs in light of its own initiatives to collect and analyzes samples of food products for microbial and chemical contaminants and infectious and toxic agents.

As the causal role of pathogenic microorganisms in food-borne infections was increasingly recognized during the twentieth century, it became clear that there was a need to shift from organoleptic to science-based inspection to address food-borne hazards of meat and poultry. Specifically, the leading food-borne pathogens in meat and poultry (*Campylobacter, E. coli* O157:H7, and *Salmonella*) often colonize the intestines of healthy animals and are not detectable by visual inspection (Morris 2003). After FSIS was criticized for not declaring *E. coli* O157:H7 to be an adulterant of ground beef, regulations based on Hazard Analysis and Critical Control Points (HACCP) were developed, signaling a new emphasis on industry food safety responsibilities. The evolving view of meat inspection emphasizes preventing distribution of meat and poultry containing high loads of pathogens capable of affecting humans. Inspection should provide an opportunity to inform suppliers and producers of hazards and to encourage best food safety practices prior to slaughter and processing (Edwards et al. 1997), including on-farm HACCP (epidemiologic) programs to manage risk (Blaha 1999). FSIS also makes sure that all foreign meat and poultry processing plants exporting to the United States meet U.S. standards.

Agricultural Research Service

Within the Agricultural Research Service, the Food Safety Program conducts research aimed at decreasing the hazards of including pathogenic bacteria, viruses, sand parasites, chemical contaminants, mycotoxins, and naturally occurring toxins produced by plants in food and feed.

Animal and Plant Health Inspection Service

Animal and plant health have a direct impact on the quality and safety of the food we eat. The National Center for Animal Surveillance and National Veterinary Services Laboratories are components of the Animal and Plant Health Inspection Service. Together, they maintain several monitoring programs, including the National Animal Health Monitoring System, which monitors *Salmonella* levels in the live animals (while FSIS monitors the levels on the slaughtered animals) And conduct testing programs for bovine spongiform encephalopathy ("mad cow" disease), which affects cows and beef.

Economic Research Service

The Economic Research Service (ERS) informs public and private decision making on economic and policy issues related to agriculture, food, natural resources, and rural development by developing and distributing economic and other social science information and analysis. ERS analyses of food-borne disease include estimating the costs of food-borne disease, conducting benefit–cost analyses of alternative regulatory options, and analyzing the impact of information labeling on markets. The analyses are essential to risk assessments and permit policy makers to compare benefits and costs of alternative public policies. For example, the ERS's benefit–cost analysis of the 1997 USDA Pathogen Reduction/HACCP program found positive net benefits, even with small reductions in pathogen levels (see chapter 12).

Office of Risk Assessment and Cost–Benefit Analysis

The Office of Risk Assessment and Cost–Benefit Analysis (ORACBA) conducts analyses of risk relating to major regulations, those with an annual economic impact of at least $100 million in 1994 U.S. dollars. Their analyses make clear the nature of the risk, alternative ways of reducing it, reasoning that justifies the proposed rule, and a comparison of the likely costs and benefits of reducing the risk. ORACBA also provides guidance and technical assistance, coordinating risk analysis work across the USDA.

Environmental Protection Agency

The U.S. Environmental Protection Agency (EPA) licenses all pesticide products distributed in the United States and sets standards on the amount of pesticides that may remain on food. The Food Quality Protection Act requires the EPA to consider the public's overall exposure to pesticides (through food and water and in home environments) when setting the standard for pesticide use on foods made from plants, seafood, meat, and poultry. The EPA is also responsible for protecting against other environmental, chemical, and microbial contaminants in air and water that might threaten the safety of the food supply. These activities include establishment of safe drinking water standards, regulating toxic substances and wastes to prevent their entry into the environment and food chain, determining the safety of new pesticides, and setting tolerance levels for pesticide residues in foods.

Department of Commerce

National Marine Fisheries Services

The National Marine Fisheries Services, an agency in the National Oceanic and Atmospheric Administration, conducts a voluntary seafood inspection and grading program that checks mainly for quality. Seafood is the only major food source that is both "caught in the wild" and raised domestically. Quality and safety standards vary widely from country to country, and inspection of processing is a challenge because much of it takes place at sea. Mandatory regulation of seafood processing falls under the FDA's jurisdiction and applies to exporters, all foreign processors that export to the United States, and importers.

International Organizations

International bodies seek to harmonize food safety standards so that exported foods meet the equivalency requirements of the importing nation (Levitt 2001) without creating undue barriers to trade (Thiermann 2000). In 1961, the Food and Agriculture Organization (FAO) of the United Nations resolved to set up the Codex Alimentarius Commission to "protect the consumer's health, ensure quality, and reduce trade barriers" (Thiermann 2000), and in 1963 the Joint FAO/World Health Organization Food Standards Programme was established, adopting the statutes of the Codex Alimentarius Commission.

Several countries in the European Union require pathogen testing of poultry and livestock in the week prior to slaughter. The ability to predict pathogen loads on live animals makes it possible to sequence processing so that animals with low pathogen loads enter establishments at the beginning of a shift and animals with the highest pathogen loads enter immediately prior to postoperation cleaning and disinfection of the establishment (clean to dirty). This type of "risk-based" meat inspection program allows high-risk livestock to receive added attention in the abattoir. In this way, producers with herds contaminated with food-borne pathogens shoulder at least some of the added cost. In addition to permitting branding of products that meet high food safety standards, this type of inspection helps place restrictions on the disposition of animals with high pathogen loads (e.g., cooking of high-risk product before sale) (Wegener et al. 2003).

Regulation

All levels of government develop legislations, statutes, and regulations to ensure a safe food supply. Legislation refers to laws presented to a political unit vested with the power to legislate, such as the congress of a nation or state. Statutes come from legislation enacted by a legislative body of a nation or state. Regulations are governmental orders prescribed by an agency of the national, state, or local government, in accordance with and having the force of law. There are a good many statutes and regulations covering multiple points along the food-to-table continuum.

At the national level, several statutes and regulations stand out as turning points in the history of food safety regulation. Public furor over conditions in food manufacturing plants in 1906 led to the passage of food safety legislation. Over time these acts have evolved into the Federal Meat Inspection Act and the Food, Drug, and Cosmetic Act (see chapter 1). The most significant new food safety regulations of the 1990s were HACCP programs for meat, poultry (Billy and Wachsmuth 1997), seafood, and other foods (e.g., produce). Although the term "adulterated" is the statutory basis for the authority of both FSIS and the FDA, it assumes that inspectors can see, taste, or smell when food is unsafe and does not reflect the natural history of most food-borne infectious diseases. The most frequent food-borne pathogens typically have no effect on the appearance (or taste or smell) of food or health of animals and plants (Taylor 1997). They are ubiquitous in nature and are thus difficult to classify as adulterants. FSIS has succeeded in classifying *E. coli* O157 in ground beef and *Listeria* and *Salmonella* in ready-to-eat foods as adulterants, but this is an exception rather than the rule.

Enforcement

A system of laws works only if there is a way of demonstrating compliance or violation and a way to enforce compliance. Inspection, product recalls, and closures of operation (restaurants or plants) are used at various levels of government to ensure compliance with food safety laws. Above, local inspection of restaurants was described. At the national level, both FSIS and FDA inspect food processing plants to ensure compliance with federal regulations, but the specifics of their inspection systems vary with each agency. Most consumers in the United States are familiar with the USDA seal demonstrating that the meat and poultry in question have been inspected (figure 13-2).

A food recall is intended to remove food products from commerce when there is reason to believe that the products may be adulterated or misbranded. Again, recalls are carried out by various government authorities and are used throughout the world. Box 13-1 lists Canadian recalls for a three-month period between 2005 and 2006.

In the United States, recalls can take place at the federal or state level. At the federal level, both FSIS and FDA may issue food recalls. FSIS recalls are initiated by the manufacturer or distributor of the meat or poultry, sometimes at the request of FSIS, and are voluntary. However, if a company refuses to recall its products, then FSIS has the legal authority to detain and seize those products in commerce. There are four primary means by which unsafe or improperly labeled meat and poultry products come to the attention of FSIS: (1) the company that manufactured or distributed the food informs FSIS of the potential hazard; (2) test results received by FSIS as part of its monitoring program indicate that the products are adulterated or, in some situations, misbranded; (3) FSIS field inspectors and program investigators discover unsafe or improperly labeled foods; or (4) epidemiologic data submitted by state or local public health departments or other federal agencies, such as the FDA or the CDC, reveal unsafe, unwholesome, or inaccurately labeled food.

Hazard Analysis and Critical Control Points

Throughout the world, regulatory agencies have adopted variations of HACCP procedures to monitor and control production operations (as discussed in chapter 10). Food manufacturers must first identify food safety hazards and critical control points in their particular production, processing, and marketing activities. Plants must then establish critical limits, or maximum or minimum levels, for each critical control point. Each plant must list procedures for monitoring the critical limits to ensure that they are met and the frequency of

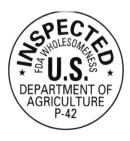

Figure 13-2. Most consumers who shop in the United States are familiar with the USDA seal found on meats and meat products in the supermarket, but many do not realize that the seal represents a complex system of inspections and regulations aimed to protect the consumer.

BOX 13-1

Governments throughout the world have varying types of authority to request or demand food recall when foods endanger the public health. Governments also take steps to provide information about recalls to the public. Below is an example of announcements of food recalls by the Canadian Food Inspection Agency.

Canadian Food Inspection Agency   **Agence canadienne d'inspection des aliments**

Canada

Food Recalls and Allergy Alerts

February 2006

- February 10—ALLERGY ALERT—Undeclared soy in LONDON PORTUGUESE BAKERY brand BREAD and BREAD PRODUCTS
- February 3—EXPANDED HEALTH HAZARD ALERT—Certain AQUAFUCHSIA brand SPROUTS may contain Salmonella bacteria
- February 2—HEALTH HAZARD ALERT—Certain AQUAFUCHSIA brand SPROUTS may contain Salmonella bacteria

January 2006

- January 27—ALLERGY ALERT—Undeclared peanut protein in YOGOURT RAISINS prepared for JOHNVINCE FOODS
- January 19—ALLERGY ALERT—Undeclared wheat in MERIT SELECTION GARDEN AND SALAD 10-CUT WEDGE POTATOES
- January 11—ALLERGY ALERT—Undeclared egg protein in PICCOLI FIORETTI ITALIAN BAKERY CRANBERRY ORANGE COFFEE CAKE

December 2005

- December 24—HEALTH HAZARD ALERT—Mung Bean Sprouts manufactured by TORONTO SUN WAH TRADING may contain Salmonella bacteria
- December 22—HEALTH HAZARD WARNING—Health Canada warns consumers not to take products containing chaparral

their monitoring activities. HACCP also includes steps for record keeping and verification.

Under HACCP, companies determine which hazards are reasonably likely to occur on their products (based largely on epidemiologic and microbiologic surveillance), where in their operation those hazards are most likely to be introduced, what controls will effectively limit the hazards, and what type of monitoring is needed to ensure that the system is working properly. Performance standards enable regulatory agencies to verify that HACCP procedures are working as intended. These standards serve as a floor to assure that producers comply with food safety regulatory expectations (Morris 2003).

The 1990s-era HACCP regulations were designed to clarify the responsibilities of industry for food safety and delineate the government's oversight role. Under HACCP, for example, FSIS no longer assumes lead responsibility for approving blueprints, equipment, and establishment sanitation. Establishment managers are responsible for deciding how an establishment operates. Agency inspectors verify that a company's HACCP plan is appropriate and that the company meets food safety performance standards. This approach delineates responsibilities based on what people do best: companies seek to produce a safe product, and government provides oversight and enforcement to protect public health.

HACCP is an iterative process that changes in response to new hazards and controls. In the years since HACCP was implemented for meat, poultry, and seafood, some gaps have been identified in implementation. Some producers embraced HACCP, while others lagged behind or appeared to "go through the motions." Only a few establishments have no HACCP plan; however, some HACCP plans do not reflect every step in the process. Other plans fail to recognize hazards that are likely to occur or do not identify control points for a stated hazard. In 2001, the FDA instituted a mid-course correction to its seafood HACCP program to focus on the producers that pose elevated risk to consumers (Levitt 2001). Around the same time, FSIS began in-depth verification of beef grinding and slaughter facilities that could present a particular *E. coli* O157:H7 hazard to consumers, assessments in poultry establishments with elevated *Salmonella* prevalence, and establishments that produce ready-to-eat foods with *Listeria monocytogenes* contamination.

Epidemiologic Data, Regulation, and Enforcement

Law making is often compared to sausage making, and in the case of food safety, law making is about sausage making (and other processes). If nothing else, food safety regulations are complex, requiring coordination between multiple levels of government and many different interests within government.

Since everyone eats food, and almost no one grows all their own food, in the United States or anywhere in the world, every person has a stake in safe food. And since almost everyone buys some portion of their food supply, every consumer has a stake in food being affordable, and thus a stake in minimizing the costs of a safe food supply. Farmers, manufacturers, retailers, and restaurant owners may be most aware of the financial costs of food safety measures (and the regulations requiring those measures), but consumers benefit when food is inexpensive. Careful analysis of the many factors contributing to food-borne illness permits thoughtful and effective regulations and a minimal impact on the cost of food. It is a challenge to bring epidemiologic data and principles to the worldwide debates on food ingredients (genetically modified) or risks ("mad cow" disease) and an environment in which the voice of science is often muted amidst competing claims from many different directions—restaurateurs earning their livelihoods, food preparers working without the benefit of paid sick leave, international bans on the import or export of an agricultural product, and everything else in between.

In most areas of public health where epidemiology is applied, epidemiologic data and studies are used to inform discussions and general debate over policy issues. Only rarely does one epidemiological study initiate a specific action; more typically, studies are repeated in different populations and settings, and the weight of the evidence is viewed in the context of other bodies of knowledge such as molecular biology, cell physiology, virology, immunology, and the like (generally referred to as biologic plausibility). In contrast to this cumulative evidence model, food-borne outbreaks are investigated one time only, and the results of the investigation may spur food safety agencies to initiate regulatory actions such as product recalls (figure 13-3), consumer advisories, or plant closures. This is a challenge both for regulators who need to understand the epidemiological evidence, and for epidemiologists whose investigation may become the basis for legal action. A clash of intellectual cultures can ensue, with regulators expecting clarity, definitive results, and quantitative criteria for evaluating an epidemiologic study. At present, there is some debate over the use of epidemiologic data in regulatory actions, and this is probably the beginning, rather than the middle or end, of discussion about applying epidemiologic data to food safety responsibilities.

The role of epidemiology in food-safety risk assessment and rule making is more familiar to epidemiologists, as it is analogous to the role of epidemiology in environmental risk assessment. It might rely on a body of evidence that is considered in light of other types of information. Even so, regulators are concerned about the use of epidemiologic data, evaluation of ambiguous results, data quality, and uncertainty around estimates. In this latter use, epidemiologic methods are well developed but may not have been fully applied or fully understood by the policy makers interested using the information. The

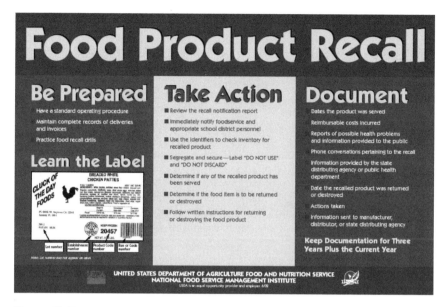

Figure 13-3. The USDA and the National Food Service Management Institute prepared this poster to help educate businesses in the food industry about food product recalls. Source: USDA.

pressures and expectations on epidemiology in the area of food safety policy are great. The opportunities to benefit the public are also great. Application of epidemiologic principles to problems of food safety should produce valuable information that can lead to more effective prevention and control of food-borne illness.

References

Billy, T. J., and I. K. Wachsmuth. (1997). "Hazard analysis and critical control point systems in the United States Department of Agriculture regulatory policy." *Rev Sci Tech* 16(2): 342–348.

Blaha, T. (1999). "Epidemiology and quality assurance application to food safety." *Prev Vet Med* 39(2): 81–92.

Carr, C. J., and F. C. Lu. (1998). "Partnership for food safety education—'Fight BAC!'" *Regul Toxicol Pharmacol* 27(3): 281–282.

Federal Food, Drug, and Cosmetic Act. 21 USC, Chapter 9, Section 301 et seq.

Federal Food Quality Protection Act (FQPA) Public Law 104–170, Aug. 3, 1906

Federal Meat Inspection Act. 21 USC, Chapter 12, Section 601 et seq.

Federal Poultry Products Inspection Act 21 USC, chapter 10, Section 451 et seq.

Levitt, J. A. (2001). "FDA's foods program." *Food Drug Law J* 56(3): 255–266.

Morris, J. G., Jr. (2003). "The color of hamburger: slow steps toward the development of a science-based food safety system in the United States." *Trans Am Clin Climatol Assoc* 114: 191–202.

Sobel, J., A. B. Hirshfeld, et al. (2000). "The pandemic of *Salmonella* Enteritidis phage type 4 reaches Utah: a complex investigation confirms the need for continuing rigorous control measures." *Epidemiol Infect* 125(1): 1–8.

Taylor, M. R. (1997). "Preparing America's food safety system for the twenty-first century —who is responsible for what when it comes to meeting the food safety challenges of the consumer-driven global economy?" *Food Drug Law J* 52(1): 13–30.

Thiermann, A. B. (2000). "Protecting health, facilitating trade, or both?" *Ann N Y Acad Sci* 916: 24–30.

Tilden, J., Jr., W. Young, et al. (1996). "A new route of transmission for *Escherichia coli*: infection from dry fermented salami." *Am J Public Health* 86(8 pt 1): 1142–1145.

Tollefson, L., F. J. Angulo, et al. (1998). "National surveillance for antibiotic resistance in zoonotic enteric pathogens." *Vet Clin North Am Food Anim Pract* 14(1): 141–150.

Wegener, H. C., T. Hald, et al. (2003). "Salmonella control programs in Denmark." *Emerg Infect Dis* 9(7): 774–780.

INDEX

Page numbers followed by "t" denote tables, "b" boxes, and "f" figures.

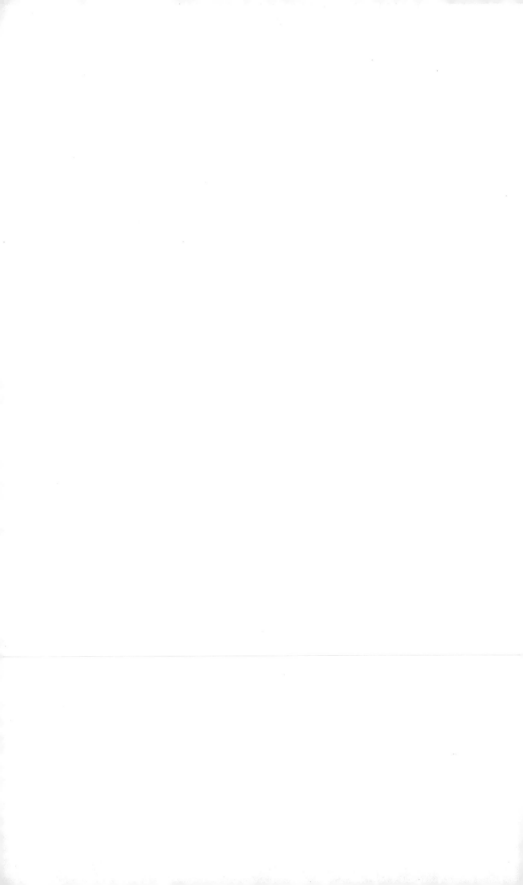